# Physical Comorbidities of Dementia

# Physical Comorbidities of Dementia

## Susan Kurrle

Curran Chair in Health Care of Older People, The Faculty of Medicine,
University of Sydney, Sydney, and Geriatrician and Clinical Director,
Division of Rehabilitation and Aged Care, Hornsby Ku-ring-gai Health Service,
Hornsby, NSW, Australia

## Henry Brodaty

Scientia Professor of Ageing and Mental Health and Director,
The Dementia Collaborative Research Centre,
University of New South Wales, Sydney, NSW, and Director,
Aged Care Psychiatry at Prince of Wales Hospital, Randwick,
Sydney, NSW, Australia

## Roseanne Hogarth

Clinical Nurse Consultant in Dementia,
Hornsby Ku-ring-gai Hospital, Sydney,
NSW, Australia

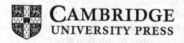

CAMBRIDGE
UNIVERSITY PRESS

# CAMBRIDGE
## UNIVERSITY PRESS

University Printing House, Cambridge CB2 8BS, United Kingdom

One Liberty Plaza, 20th Floor, New York, NY 10006, USA

477 Williamstown Road, Port Melbourne, VIC 3207, Australia

314-321, 3rd Floor, Plot 3, Splendor Forum, Jasola District Centre, New Delhi - 110025, India

79 Anson Road, #06-04/06, Singapore 079906

Cambridge University Press is part of the University of Cambridge.

It furthers the University's mission by disseminating knowledge in the pursuit of education, learning and research at the highest international levels of excellence.

www.cambridge.org
Information on this title: www.cambridge.org/9781107648265

First published 2012

*A catalogue record for this publication is available from the British Library*

*Library of Congress Cataloging in Publication data*
Kurrle, Susan.
   Physical comorbidities of dementia / Susan Kurrle, Henry Brodaty, Roseanne Hogarth.
     p. ; cm.
   Includes bibliographical references and index.
   ISBN 978-1-107-64826-5 (pbk.)
   I. Brodaty, Henry.   II. Hogarth, Roseanne.   III. Title.
   [DNLM: 1. Dementia–complications.   2. Dementia–physiopathology.
   3. Dementia–therapy. WM 220]
   616.8´3–dc23
   2012013673

ISBN 978-1-107-64826-5 Paperback

................................................................................................

# Contents

| | | |
|---|---|---|
| *Foreword* | | *page* vi |
| *Preface* | | ix |
| 1 | Introduction | 1 |
| 2 | Falls | 3 |
| 3 | Delirium | 15 |
| 4 | Epilepsy | 30 |
| 5 | Weight loss and nutritional disorders | 40 |
| 6 | Incontinence | 60 |
| 7 | Sleep disturbance | 74 |
| 8 | Visual dysfunction | 86 |
| 9 | Oral disease | 99 |
| 10 | Frailty | 111 |
| *Index* | | 120 |

# Foreword

Less than a third of people over the age of 55 years suffer from only one disease when ill; two-thirds will have at least one other disease. Comorbidity – particularly in advanced age – is becoming the rule rather than the exception. And yet, health systems, even in highly developed countries, are not organized in a manner that would provide appropriate care for people with more than one illness. This is particularly true for the comorbidity of mental and physical illness, but it also holds for the care of people with more than one physical illness, who receive suboptimal care in health systems that are increasingly often fragmented into superspecialties. The neglect of comorbidity leads to higher levels of disability and poorer prognosis for the comorbid conditions. The cost of care when only one of the comorbid conditions is given attention is much higher, mainly because of complications that could have been avoided if all comorbid conditions had been treated at the same time. In developing countries the situation is even worse, partly because of restricted resources but also because of the lesser competence of dealing with mental disorders consequent to the low priority given to mental disorders and psychiatry in the education of health personnel.

These considerations have led the Association for the Improvement of Mental Health (AMH) Programme to initiate several projects aiming to increase the awareness of all concerned about the high prevalence of comorbidity and about the importance of making arrangements that will allow its appropriate management. One of these projects aims to provide reviews of evidence and experience about comorbidity. This book, *Physical Comorbidities of Dementia* is the most recent of the reviews whose production the Association has stimulated – the previous reviews dealt with physical illness and schizophrenia (Leucht et al.), intellectual disability and ill Health (O'Hara, McCarthy and Bouras) and physical illness and drugs of abuse (Gordon). We hope that these books will be read widely, and we plan to have them translated and published in languages other than English.

I am delighted to see this book in print, because I believe that it will help to give the problem of comorbidity of dementia and physical illness the attention that it deserves. The way in which the authors approached this issue is innovative and different from the approaches that were used in the other reviews mentioned above: rather than presenting the comorbidity between diseases the book examines the impact that a particular feature of several other diseases might have on care that should be offered to people with dementia. This way of approaching the problem will be very useful to the specialists in geriatrics and psychiatry, to general practitioners, nurses, and other personnel, as well as to nonprofessional carers: it is, however, also a novel way of approaching issues related to care and might therefore be of interest and applicable in the development of reviews and guidelines concerning comorbidity. I take pleasure in recommending this book to all those concerned with the care of older people.

Professor Norman Sartorius
President
Association for the Improvement of Mental Health Programmes (AMH)
14 chemin Colladon
1209 Geneva
Switzerland

# Preface

This book began life as a brief literature review after two of the authors had a discussion about the physical conditions that are more commonly seen in people with dementia than in the general population. It was aided in its development by patients and carers who reported unusual symptoms that were not adequately explained by conventional knowledge on dementia. These symptoms included seizures masquerading as falls, distorted vision, and difficulty recognizing familiar objects, as well as unexplained weight loss despite eating well. A wide-ranging review of the literature uncovered nine physical conditions that occur more often in people with dementia. When the authors were invited by Professor Norman Sartorius to contribute a book to the series on comorbidity of mental and physical illness that his Association was organizing, they turned their review into the book that is presented here.

Of concern to the authors is that despite the increasing numbers of people with dementia, a lack of knowledge exists about the health conditions, such as epilepsy, that occur more commonly in people with dementia. While there has been a great deal of focus on the cognitive and behavioral symptoms of dementia and their management, the physical comorbidities of dementia have been neglected. These comorbidities, which include delirium, seizures, visual dysfunction, incontinence, and sleep disorders, are common and impact greatly on the care and quality of life of the person with dementia, their caregivers, and family members. As many of these physical conditions are treatable, appropriate recognition and treatment are likely to reduce disability and improve quality of life.

This book is designed for medical practitioners, nurses, and allied health staff working with people with dementia. It fills a major gap in knowledge by providing a comprehensive overview of the health-related scientific literature on many of the physical conditions that accompany and complicate dementia. It describes how these conditions may present, and what the underlying pathology is likely to be, and gives detailed information and evidence-based recommendations on how to recognize and manage these conditions. The book aims to provide practical explanations and suggestions on improving care for people with dementia.

The literature review was funded by the Australian Government through the Dementia Collaborative Research Centre program, and by the Curran Ageing Research Unit at Hornsby Ku-ring-gai Hospital, Sydney. The authors wish to thank Jennifer Hill for her work in searching the literature and developing outlines for several of the chapters, and Racheal de Gabriele for her initial assistance in reviewing the literature. Professor Norman Sartorius provided encouragement and advice in developing this book, and his assistance is gratefully acknowledged. Finally our patients and their carers deserve special thanks for providing the inspiration and the impetus for this book.

# Introduction

This book describes the physical health conditions (physical comorbidities) that occur more commonly in people with dementia than in the general population. A **comorbidity** is defined as a disease or condition that coexists with another disease. The physical comorbidities of dementia that have been identified and are investigated in this review of the literature are:

- falls
- delirium
- weight loss and malnutrition
- epilepsy
- frailty
- sleep disorders
- oral disease
- visual dysfunction
- incontinence.

## Method

Using the search term "exp dementia" in MEDLINE (1966–2011), articles on physical comorbidities of dementia were identified from the medical, nursing, and psychological literature. For each physical comorbidity, specific search terms were used and then combined using Boolean techniques. Results were then restricted using the tags "human" and "English language," and then restricted further by date to those published after 1990. All abstracts from these articles were reviewed and the results were further confined to peer-reviewed publications, to exclude less robust findings. Reference lists from these articles were hand-searched for further references.

## Results

A total of 2512 full articles was obtained, and information was extracted and summarized using the one page JAPICO (Journal, Authors, Participants, Interventions, Comparisons, Outcomes) summary method. The search covered the literature up to 2011. The information has been summarized for each comorbidity in separate chapters, and recommendations have been developed based on the available evidence. The literature has not been graded according to the level of scientific evidence, but the type of study from which the information has been obtained is described in the text, and all references are provided at the end of each chapter.

# Falls

## Introduction

A fall is defined as an event reported by the faller or a witness, resulting in a person inadvertently coming to rest on the ground or another lower level (Shaw, 2002). Falls are a major health issue in older people, with more than 30% of those aged 65 and over reporting a fall in the previous year (AGS et al., 2001). A single fall may precipitate a downward spiral of immobility, reduced confidence and incapacity, eventually resulting in early institutionalization and death (Rowe and Fehrenbach, 2004, AGS and BGS, 2011). Studies have consistently shown that dementia is associated with an increased risk of falls, at a rate at least twice that of cognitively intact older people, with an annual incidence of falls in people with dementia of 70–80% (van Doorn et al., 2003, Allan et al., 2009). The risk of hip fracture is also increased in this population group (Weller and Schatzker, 2004), and people with dementia recover less well after a fall than those without the disease (Shaw, 2002).

## Epidemiology of falls in dementia

Early studies by Campbell et al. (1981), Buchner and Larson (1987) and Tinetti et al. (1988) showed that falls were far more common in people with cognitive impairment and dementia than in those without dementia. Indeed, Tinetti and colleagues found that cognitive impairment led to a 5-fold increase in falls in a prospective 1-year study of 336 community-dwelling older people. Van Dijk et al. (1993) reported a falls rate of 4 falls per patient per year in a 2-year study of 240 nursing home patients with dementia. A prospective cohort study with 2 years' follow-up of more than 2000 nursing home residents also found a falls rate of 4 falls per patient per year, compared with 2.3 falls per year among residents without dementia, showing that dementia conferred a relative risk of 1.74 for falling (van Doorn et al., 2003). In a cross-sectional study of 2008 older residents in geriatric care settings who were cognitively impaired, Kallin et al. (2005) found that 9.4%

had fallen in the previous week. In a prospective study of cognitively impaired older people presenting to an emergency department with a fall, 77% of the overall group fell during the 1-year follow-up period (Shaw et al., 2003). In a prospective community-based longitudinal study of older people with an 8-year period of follow-up, Anstey et al. (2006) found a strong association between decreasing cognitive function and an increasing risk of falls. In a prospective study of 140 people with dementia and 39 healthy controls, Allan and colleagues (2009) demonstrated an 8-fold increase in falls in people with dementia over a 1-year period compared with healthy controls.

Not only are people with cognitive impairment and dementia more likely to fall, but they are also more susceptible to injuries when falling (Oleske et al., 1995, Kallin et al., 2005). Sustaining a fall was the leading reason for acute hospital admission in a 3-year prospective cohort study of 827 community-dwelling older people with dementia (Rudolph et al., 2010). People with cognitive impairment are more likely to sustain a serious injury, with the annual incidence of fractures being approximately 7%, compared with a 3% annual incidence in the older population generally (Buchner and Larson, 1987, Campbell et al., 1990). In a 1-year prospective study of 112 people over the age of 55 years with dementia and 100 control subjects, Asada et al. (1996) found that 41% of the people with dementia suffered a fall-related injury, compared with only 11% of the controls. Dementia is also associated with a 3- to 4-fold increase in the risk of hip fractures and a 3-fold increase in the 6-month post-fracture mortality rate compared with older people without dementia (Vidan et al., 2005). Fall-related injuries resulting in hospitalization are important determining factors in the discharge destination of patients with dementia. In a review of 153 hospitalized patients, Rowe and Fehrenbach (2004) found that 65% of community-dwelling patients with dementia who were admitted following a fall-related injury were later discharged to institutional care, rather than returning to their pre-admission domicile.

Several studies have shown that falls are most likely to occur in those people with moderately severe dementia who are still mobile but may need help to rise from a chair, or need a helper or a walking aid (Nakamura et al., 1996, Kallin et al., 2005). Once a person's dementia is sufficiently severe to require bed confinement, a fall is no longer likely to occur.

## Etiology of falls in dementia

In the general population, the risk of falling is determined by numerous factors. These include a previous history of falls, impairments of balance, muscle strength, coordination and gait, impaired vision, functional impairment, medical conditions of the heart or brain causing fainting or low blood pressure, medication use, impaired cognition and mood, environmental hazards, and inappropriate footwear (AGS et al., 2001). These factors are all relevant to patients with dementia. In addition, there are many other possible reasons why people with cognitive impairment or dementia have an increased risk of falls, and a systematic review of prospective studies by Harlein et al. (2009) identified disease-specific motor impairments, the type and severity of dementia suffered, behavioral disturbances, neuroleptic medication, and low bone mineral density as being additional risk factors for falls in dementia.

## Gait impairment in dementia

Gait and balance abnormalities are seen commonly in dementia, particularly in people with vascular dementia, diffuse Lewy body disease (DLBD), and Parkinson's disease with dementia. Similarly, a cautious gait pattern with decreased step length and height, variability in stride length, a reduced arm swing and cadence, and a flexed posture is commonly seen in Alzheimer's disease (AD) (Allan et al., 2005, Webster et al., 2006). Impairments in coordination and balance have been shown in older people with cognitive impairment and mild AD (Franssen et al., 1999), and greater stride length variability has been shown to be associated with a higher risk of falls (Nakamura et al., 1996). Waite and colleagues (2000) examined motor performance in 92 older people with dementia, and found that people with Parkinson's disease with dementia had the poorest performance, although gait abnormalities were also seen in all other types of dementia. They suggested that the gait abnormalities seen in people with Parkinson's disease with dementia were related to pathology in the substantia nigra, and to white matter ischemia in vascular dementia. In a study of 210 older people with dementia who had presented to the emergency department with a fall, 99% were found to have an impairment of gait or balance (Shaw et al., 2003).

Normal walking has been shown to require not only intact motor and sensory systems, but also intact executive control, navigational and visuospatial abilities, and attention, in order to choose an appropriate path while recognizing and avoiding hazards (Snijders et al., 2007). Good postural stability is also important for normal walking – thus poor control of postural sway, inadequate vision, and increased reaction times can all contribute to an increased risk of falling (Lord et al., 1996). Dementia can affect all of these abilities, leading to an increased risk of falling when these functions are affected. The hippocampal area of the brain is affected early in AD, and it has been shown to play a role not only in cognition, but also in gait, with functions related to the orientation of the body in space. It has been postulated that degeneration in the hippocampus causes gait disturbances as well as memory problems in people with AD (Scherder et al., 2007). A disintegration of higher cortical sensory functions in AD, including the visuospatial integration that is necessary for a motor function such as walking, has also been suggested as a reason for impaired gait and postural control (Sheridan and Hausdorff, 2007). Additionally, those with dementia may have an unrealistic perception of their own motor abilities, resulting in impulsivity and risk-taking behavior, which also contributes to the risk of falling.

## Dementia pathology

A reduced ability to perform more than one task at one time (known as dual tasking or multitasking) has been shown to predict falls risk in older people (Lundin-Olsson et al., 1998). Dementia is associated with reduced attention and the subsequent inability to perform more than one task adequately at a time. Using the dual task "talking while walking" test, Camicioli and colleagues (1997) showed slowing in the walking speed of people with dementia while performing this task, compared with older people without dementia, which they suggested may increase the risk of falls in this group. Similar findings were reported by Hauer and colleagues (2003), who compared dual tasking in younger people and older people with and without dementia, and found a marked reduction in motor performance in the subjects with dementia while dual tasking. Pettersson and colleagues (2007) demonstrated that this also occurred in people with cognitive impairment or dementia under the age of 65, with a decreased walking speed observed during the dual task test.

Neurovascular instability, a condition involving orthostatic hypotension, vaso-vagal syncope, and carotid sinus hypersensitivity, is a known risk factor for falls in the general population, and is also considered an important factor in the occurrence of falls in older people with dementia. Compared with cognitively intact older people, neurovascular instability shows increased prevalence in people with dementia, with orthostatic hypotension reported in up to 40% of older people with dementia (Shaw and Kenny, 2001), and carotid hypersensitivity in 28% of AD patients compared with 41% of people with DLBD (Ballard et al., 1999). Postural hypotension is commonly seen in people with DLBD and Parkinson's disease with dementia, and was shown to be a significant risk factor for falls in a 1-year prospective study of 179 older people with mild to moderate dementia (Allan et al., 2009).

## Effects of medication

Centrally active medications such as antipsychotics, antidepressants, and benzo-diazepines are well known to increase the risk of falls in the population generally (Tinetti et al., 1988, Campbell et al., 1989, Leipzig et al., 1999). Given that these medications are commonly prescribed in people with dementia, the risk of falls is concurrently increased. Buchner and Larson (1987) noted the high number of falls associated with psychotropic drug prescriptions, and in a 1-year study of 124 people with AD, Horikawa and colleagues (2005) showed a 3-fold increase in falls associated with the administration of neuroleptic drugs. In their large study of 2008 older people with cognitive impairment, Kallin and colleagues (2005) showed that the risk of falls increased with the specific serotonin reuptake inhibitors, and with the atypical antipsychotic drug olanzapine. Although Asada et al. (1996) found some increased risk of falls with psychotropic medication, this association did not reach statistical significance. Tangman et al. (2010) found that the adverse effects of neuroleptics and benzodiazepines were the cause in more than half of falls occurring in a psychogeriatric hospital. This increased risk for falls may relate to the effects of psychotropic medications on balance and reaction time, as well as heightening risk through postural hypotension, extrapyramidal side effects, and increased sedation (Shaw and Kenny, 2001).

Cholinesterase inhibitors are used as symptomatic treatment in AD and other dementias, and various studies have shown them to increase the risk of syncope and hip fracture in some older people (Gill et al., 2009). However, Kallin and colleagues (2005) did not find any association between the cholinesterase inhibitors and falls in their large study. A meta-analysis of randomized trials of the cholinesterase inhibitors and memantine, also used as a symptomatic treatment in AD, showed that the cholinesterase inhibitors may increase the chance of syncope in patients, but were not directly associated with an increased risk for falls or fractures (Kim et al., 2011).

## Behavioral disturbances

Behavioral disturbances, and in particular a tendency for wandering, were identified by Buchner and Larson (1987) as contributing to falls risk in 157 older people with dementia. Resistance to care, apathy, and wandering contributed to an increased risk for falls and fall-related injuries in a study of 112 people with dementia, reported by Asada and colleagues (1996). Kallin and colleagues (2005) found that wandering, verbal disruption, attention-seeking behavior and restlessness were significantly associated with falls – as were hyperactive, paranoid, depressive, and hallucinatory symptoms. It would seem that many of these symptoms are associated with increased physical activity, leading to an increased chance of falling.

There is some evidence that the type of dementia is likely to affect the risk of falls. Ballard et al. (1999) showed that falls were more common in patients with DLBD than in AD; a finding supported by Imamura and colleagues (2000), whose prospective study of 561 patients with dementia also reflected these relative rates of falls between the dementia types. Similar results were found in the prospective study by Allan and colleagues (2009), in which falls were much more common in people with a diagnosis of DLBD and Parkinson's disease with dementia than in AD. In a 6-month study of 110 older subjects with dementia, Kanemura and colleagues (2000) found that patients with vascular dementia were twice as likely to fall as those patients with AD.

In a study designed to examine precipitating factors (rather than risk factors) for falls among dementia patients, Tangman and colleagues (2010) prospectively examined the circumstances surrounding falls occurring in older patients in a psychogeriatric hospital ward over a 2-year period. They found that the acute onset of disease and acute drug side effects were the precipitating factors accounting for the majority of the falls, with delirium and urinary tract infections implicated in one-quarter of falls. A smaller number of falls were caused by interactions with others, particularly being pushed over by another person.

## Management of falls and falls risk in people with cognitive impairment and dementia

### Assessment

A multifactorial assessment for falls risk is recommended for all older people who have had a fall or have gait or balance problems (AGS and BGS, 2011). As people with dementia are at increased risk of falls, it is likely that most will have had a fall in the previous year (Shaw et al., 2003). Thus an assessment of risk factors for each individual may reveal areas where risk is heightened and where modifications can be made to mitigate this risk. This assessment should include: the circumstances surrounding falls that have occurred; current medications, focusing particularly on those known to increase falls risk (including psychotropics and antihypertensives); an evaluation of gait and balance, muscle strength, heart rate and rhythm, and blood pressure and the presence of postural hypotension; and a review of footwear and environmental hazards. The presence of urinary incontinence has also been shown to be a risk factor for falls. Delbaere and colleagues (2008) suggested testing older people for their ability to stand unaided, including on a foam mat, as a key indicator of falls risk for those in residential care.

### Interventions

There is strong evidence supporting interventions to prevent falls in the older population generally, but no studies have been successful in showing that falls can be prevented in people with dementia. There is also considered to be insufficient evidence to support any recommendations that aim to reduce falls risk in older people with cognitive impairment (AGS and BGS, 2011). Shaw and colleagues (2003) trialed a multifactorial assessment and intervention to prevent falls in older people with cognitive impairment or dementia after they presented to an emergency department following a fall. They found no significant effect associated with the intervention (which had been effective in a cognitively intact population), and suggested that this lack of effect may be due to different causal pathways for falls in people with dementia compared with the general population.

Studies in residential-care facilities have indicated that multifactorial interventions may be effective in preventing or reducing falls in a population of frail older people, some of whom have dementia (Feder et al., 2000). Rapp and colleagues (2008) reported a trial of a multifactorial fall-prevention program involving staff and resident education, advice on environmental modifications, recommendations for hip protectors, and progressive balance and resistance training in 725 nursing home residents. They showed a significant reduction in falls in the intervention group, and also found that this effect was much greater in those residents with cognitive impairment. Conversely, however, in a similar multifactorial fall-prevention program in residential-care facilities that included staff education, environmental modifications, physical exercise, review of medications, provision of appropriate aids, and provision of hip protectors, Jensen and colleagues (2003) showed no significant reduction in falls in those residents with lower levels of cognition.

There are other interventions that have been reported to be successful in people with cognitive impairment. A cluster-randomized trial of a single intervention using staff-oriented training in residential-care facilities has been reported as showing a reduction in falls in the intervention group, with no marked difference observed between residents with and without cognitive impairment (Bouwen et al., 2008). Physical restraints are often used in hospitals and residential-care facilities in order to prevent a person with dementia from standing up or walking around, theoretically to prevent falls. However, the removal of physical restraints has not been shown to increase the occurrence of falls in older people with dementia in residential care (Capezuti, 2004), and the use of physical restraints (and in particular trunk restraints) has actually been shown to significantly increase the risk of falls in people with dementia in residential-care facilities (Luo et al., 2011).

It may be possible to extrapolate the evidence for interventions to reduce falls from the general population to apply to people with dementia. Although the American Geriatrics Society/British Geriatrics Society Clinical Practice Guideline for Prevention of Falls in Older Persons does not support this notion (AGS and BGS, 2011), and Shaw (2007) notes that the cognitively impaired population who fall may be very different from the cognitively intact older population, it seems reasonable to intervene opportunistically, and offer interventions as appropriate for each individual to reduce falls and fall-related injuries. Medication management and a reduction in psychotropic medication dosages, strength and balance training, treating any postural hypotension, treating low vitamin D levels, osteoporosis, and cataracts, conducting an occupational therapy home hazard assessment, using hip protectors and helmets, and installing fall alarms are some of the interventions that have been shown to reduce falls or fall-related injuries in the older population, and may also have transferrable use in reducing falls in older people with dementia (van Doorn et al., 2003).

Hill and colleagues (2009) suggest that to reduce falls in older people with dementia living in the community, exercise programs must incorporate movement combinations that challenge the balance system, rather than just including cardiovascular or strengthening exercises. Because it may be difficult for people in the more advanced stages of dementia to participate in complex exercise programs, they suggest targeting these programs only at those with mild to moderate dementia. However, Mirolsky-Scala and Kraemer (2009) describe a case in which an individualized balance and strengthening exercise program was developed for an older person with moderately severe dementia, taking into account her poor cognition and behavioral problems. The program resulted in clinically significant improvements in functional outcomes, and in particular her balance, illustrating the potential benefits of an individualized program in more severely affected patients. Similarly, a small study of 20 older people with dementia has shown that a physical training program to improve balance can significantly improve mobility and static balance in the intervention group, although falls were not measured (Toulotte et al., 2003).

## Recommendations

1. Consider opportunistic screening for risk modification, although no current evidence shows that screening people with dementia for falls risk is effective in reducing their fall rate.
2. Remove any physical restraints, as their use is likely to worsen the risk of falls.
3. Although no interventions are proven to prevent falls specifically in people with dementia, consider:
    a. reviewing medications, particularly psychotropics
    b. assessing and treating postural hypotension
    c. assessing and treating visual impairment due to cataracts or refraction errors
    d. treating osteoporosis and vitamin D deficiency.
4. Consider introducing the use of:
    a. exercise, particularly strength and balance training
    b. occupational therapy home hazard assessment and environmental modification
    c. hip protectors
    d. falls alarms.

---

### Case studies

Mr. E is an 84-year-old man in a dementia-specific residential aged care facility. He has moderately severe dementia and requires prompting or supervision with most activities of daily living. He loves to walk around the facility and in the gardens, but is very impulsive and has often fallen and is at risk of injuring himself. He was assessed by a physiotherapist experienced in aged care and given some simple daily balance and strengthening exercises (standing on one leg and tandem stance, and rising from a chair without using his arms) to be supervised by facility staff. Mr. E was provided with hip protectors and a light football headguard, both of which he was happy to wear as he had played rugby in his youth. A walking frame was tried but not considered appropriate as he would forget to use it. He is now falling much less often and has sustained no injuries other than mild abrasions.

Mrs. F is a 68-year-old woman who lives with her husband in their own home. She has moderate AD, as well as hypertension and coronary artery disease with a recent myocardial infarct. She is on several antihypertensive medications, and an atypical antipsychotic medication as she had been becoming somewhat aggressive. Her husband reported that she had fallen a number of times over the past 2 months, particularly after getting up in the morning, when using the toilet, and when getting out of the car. She was found to have a significant drop in her blood pressure from sitting down to standing up, and her antihypertensive medications were reduced. Her antipsychotic medication was reduced but her aggressive behavior worsened, so it was resumed at the previous dose. Mrs. F was also noted to have a very low vitamin D level and was consequently commenced on vitamin D capsules (initially 4000 IU/day) to improve this level. She was encouraged to increase her walking, and began going to the nearby park with her husband to walk on a daily basis. She has had only one fall in the 3 months following these interventions, and has also become less aggressive.

---

## Key points

- Falls occur in people with dementia at twice the rate of the normal population, and 70–80% of people with dementia will fall at least once a year.
- Fractures are three times more common in people with dementia than in the normal population, and hip fracture is also three times more common.
- The increased rate of falls may be due to the presence of gait abnormalities, orthostatic hypotension, postural instability, impaired executive function, and impaired visuospatial skills.
- No interventions have been shown to prevent falls specifically in people with dementia.

# References

Allan, L., Ballard, C., Burn, D., et al. (2005). Prevalence and severity of gait disorders in Alzheimer's and non-Alzheimer's dementias. *Journal of the American Geriatrics Society*, 53, 1681–1687.

Allan, L.M., Ballard, C.G., Rowan, E.N., et al. (2009). Incidence and prediction of falls in dementia: a prospective study in older people. *PLoS ONE*, 4, e5521.

American Geriatrics Society, British Geriatrics Society, American Academy of Orthopaedic Surgeons Panel on Falls Prevention. (2001). Guideline for the prevention of falls in older persons. *Journal of the American Geriatrics Society*, 49, 664–672.

American Geriatrics Society and British Geriatrics Society Panel on Prevention of Falls in Older Persons. (2011). Summary of the updated American Geriatrics Society/British Geriatrics Society Clinical Practice Guideline for Prevention of Falls in Older Persons. *Journal of the American Geriatrics Society*, 59, 148–157.

Anstey, K.J., von Sanden, C., Luszcz, M. (2006). An 8-year prospective study of the relationship between cognitive performance and falling in very old adults. *Journal of the American Geriatrics Society*, 54, 1169–1176.

Asada, T., Kariya, T., Kinoshita, T., et al. (1996). Predictors of fall-related injuries among community-dwelling elderly people with dementia. *Age & Ageing*, 25, 22–28.

Ballard, C.G., Shaw, F., Lowery, K., et al. (1999). The prevalence, assessment and associations of falls in dementia with Lewy bodies and Alzheimer's disease. *Dementia and Geriatric Cognitive Disorders*, 10, 97–103.

Bouwen, A., De Lepeleire, J., Buntinx, F. (2008). Rate of accidental falls in institutionalized older people with and without cognitive impairment halved as a result of a staff-oriented intervention. *Age & Ageing*, 37, 306–310.

Buchner, D.M. and Larson, E.B. (1987) Falls and fractures in patients with Alzheimer-type dementia. *Journal of the American Medical Association*, 257, 1492–1495.

Camicioli, R., Howieson, D., Lehman, S., et al. (1997). Talking while walking: the effect of a dual task in aging and Alzheimer's disease. *Neurology*, 48, 955–958.

Campbell, A.J., Borrie, M.J., Spears, G.F. (1989). Risk factors for falls in a community-based prospective study of people 70 years and older. *Journal of Gerontology: Medical Sciences*, 44, M112–M117.

Campbell, A.J., Borrie, M.J., Spears, G.F., et al. (1990). Circumstances and consequences of falls experienced by a community population 70 years and over during a prospective study. *Age & Ageing*, 19, 136–141.

Campbell, A.J., Reinken, J., Allan, B.C., et al. (1981). Falls in old age: a study of frequency and related clinical factors. *Age & Ageing*, 10, 264–270.

Capezuti, E. (2004). Minimising the use of restrictive devices in dementia patients at risk for falling. *Nursing Clinics of North America*, 39, 625–647.

Delbaere, K., Close, J., Menz, H., et al. (2008). Development and validation of fall risk screening tools for use in residential aged care facilities. *Medical Journal of Australia*, 189, 193–196.

Feder, G., Cryer, C., Donovan, S., et al. (2000). Guidelines for the prevention of falls in people over 65. *British Medical Journal*, 321, 1007–1011.

Franssen, E.H., Souren, L.E., Torossian, C.L., Reisberg, B. (1999). Equilibrium and limb coordination in mild cognitive impairment and mild Alzheimer's disease. *Journal of the American Geriatrics Society*, 47, 463–469.

Gill, S.S., Anderson, G.M., Fischer, H.D., et al. (2009). Syncope and its consequences in patients with dementia receiving cholinesterase inhibitors. *Archives of Internal Medicine*, 169, 867–873.

Harlein, J., Dassen, T., Halfens, R.J.G., et al. (2009). Fall risk factors in older people with dementia or cognitive impairment: a systematic review. *Journal of Advanced Nursing*, 65, 922–933.

Hauer, K., Pfisterer, M., Weber, C., et al. (2003) Cognitive impairment decreases postural control during dual tasks in geriatric patients with a history of severe falls. *Journal of the American Geriatrics Society*, 51, 1638–1644.

Hill, K.D., LoGiudice, D., Lautenschlager, N.T., et al. (2009). Effectiveness of balance training exercise in people with mild to moderate severity Alzheimer's disease: protocol for a randomized trial. *BMC Geriatrics*, 9, 29.

Horikawa, E., Matsui, T., Arai, H., et al. (2005). Risk of falls in Alzheimer's disease: a prospective study. *Internal Medicine*, 44, 717–721.

Imamura, T., Hirono, N., Hashimoto, M., et al. (2000) Fall-related injuries in dementia with Lewy bodies (DLB) and Alzheimer's disease. *European Journal of Neurology*, 7, 77–79.

Jensen, J., Nyberg, L., Gustafson, Y., et al. (2003). Fall and injury prevention in residential care-effects in residents with higher and lower levels of cognition. *Journal of the American Geriatrics Society,* 51, 627–635.

Kallin, K., Gustafson, Y., Sandman, P., et al. (2005). Factors associated with falls among older, cognitively impaired people in geriatric care settings. *American Journal of Geriatric Psychiatry,* 13, 501–509.

Kanemura, N., Kobayashi, R., Inafuku, K., et al. (2000). Analysis of risk factors for falls in the elderly with dementia. *Journal of Physical Therapy & Science,* 12, 27–31.

Kim, D.H., Brown, R.T., Ding, E.L., et al. (2011). Dementia medications and risk of falls, syncope, and related adverse events: meta-analysis of randomized controlled trials. *Journal of the American Geriatrics Society,* 59, 1019–1031.

Leipzig, R.M., Cumming, R.G., Tinetti, M.E. (1999). Drugs and falls in older people: a systematic review and meta-analysis: I. Psychotropic drugs. *Journal of the American Geriatrics Society* 47, 30–39.

Lord, S.R., Lloyd, D.G., Keung, L. S. (1996). Sensori-motor function, gait patterns and falls in community-dwelling women. *Age & Ageing,* 25, 292–299.

Lundin-Olsson, L., Nyberg, L., Gustafson, Y. (1998). Attention, frailty and falls: the effect of a manual task on basic mobility. *Journal of the American Geriatrics Society,* 46, 758–761.

Luo, H., Lin, M., Castle, N. (2011). Physical restraint use and falls in nursing homes: a comparison between residents with and without dementia. *American Journal of Alzheimer's Disease & Other Dementias,* 26, 44–50.

Mirolsky-Scala, G. and Kraemer, T. (2009). Fall management in Alzheimer-related dementia: a case study. *Journal of Geriatric Physical Therapy,* 32, 181–189.

Nakamura, T., Meguro, K., Sasaki, H. (1996). Relationship between falls and stride length variability in senile dementia of the Alzheimer type. *Gerontology,* 42, 108–113.

Oleske, D.M., Wilson, R.S., Bernard, B.A., et al. (1995). Epidemiology of injury in people with Alzheimer's disease. *Journal of the American Geriatrics Society,* 43, 741–746.

Pettersson, A.F., Olsson, E., Wahlund, L. (2007). Effect of divided attention on gait in subjects with and without cognitive impairment. *Journal of Geriatric Psychiatry and Neurology,* 20, 58–62.

Rapp, K., Lamb, S., Buchele, G., et al. (2008) Prevention of falls in nursing homes: subgroup analyses of a randomized fall prevention trial. *Journal of the American Geriatrics Society,* 56, 1092–1097.

Rowe, M.A. and Fehrenbach, M. (2004) Injuries sustained by community-dwelling individuals with dementia. *Clinical Nursing Research,* 13, 98–110.

Rudolph, J.L., Zanin, N.M., Jones, R.N., et al. (2010). Hospitalization in community-dwelling persons with Alzheimer's disease: frequency and causes. *Journal of the American Geriatrics Society,* 58, 1542–1548.

Scherder, E., Eggermont, L., Swaab, D., et al. (2007). Gait in ageing and associated dementias: its relationship with cognition. *Neuroscience and Biobehavioural Reviews,* 31, 485–497.

Shaw, F.E. (2002). Falls in cognitive impairment and dementia. *Clinics in Geriatric Medicine*, 18, 159–173.

Shaw, F.E. (2007). Prevention of falls in older people with dementia. *Journal of Neural Transmission*, 114, 1259–1264.

Shaw, F.E., Bond, J., Richardson, D.A., et al. (2003). Multifactorial intervention after a fall in older people with cognitive impairment and dementia presenting to the accident and emergency department: randomised controlled trial. *British Medical Journal*, 326, 73–79.

Shaw, F.E. and Kenny, R.A. (2001). Science of risk factors in fallers: impact of cognitive dysfunction. *Reviews in Clinical Gerontology*, 11, 299–309.

Sheridan, P.L. and Hausdorff, J.M. (2007). The role of higher-level cognitive function in gait: executive dysfunction contributes to fall risk in Alzheimer's disease. *Dementia & Geriatric Cognitive Disorders*, 24, 125–137.

Snijders, A., van de Warrenburg, B., Giladi, N., et al. (2007). Neurological gait disorders in elderly people: clinical approach and classification. *Lancet Neurology*, 6, 63–74.

Tangman, S., Eriksson, S., Gustafson, Y., et al. (2010). Precipitating factors for falls among patients with dementia on a psychogeriatric ward. *International Psychogeriatrics*, 22, 641–649.

Tinetti, M.E., Speechley, M., Ginter, S.F. (1988). Risk factors for falls among elderly persons living in the community. *New England Journal of Medicine*, 319, 1701–1707.

Toulotte, C., Fabre, C., Dangremont, B., et al. (2003). Effects of physical training on the physical capacity of frail, demented patients with a history of falling: a randomized controlled trial. *Age & Ageing*, 32, 67–73.

van Dijk, P., Meulenberg, O., van de Sande, H., et al. (1993). Falls in dementia patients. *The Gerontologist*, 33, 200–204.

van Doorn, C., Gruber-Baldini, AL., Zimmerman, S., et al. (2003). Dementia as a risk factor for falls and fall injuries among nursing home residents. *Journal of the American Geriatrics Society*, 51, 1213–1218.

Vidan, M., Serra, J.A., Moreno, C., et al. (2005). Efficacy of a comprehensive geriatric intervention in older patients hospitalized for hip fracture: a randomized controlled trial. *Journal of the American Geriatrics Society*, 53, 1476–1482.

Waite, L., Broe, G., Grayson, D., et al. (2000) Motor function and disability in the dementias. *International Journal of Geriatric Psychiatry*, 15, 897–903.

Webster, K.E., Merory, J.R., Wittwer, J.E. (2006). Gait variability in community dwelling adults with Alzheimer Disease. *Alzheimer Disease & Associated Disorders*, 20, 37–40.

Weller, I., Schatzker, J. (2004). Hip fractures and Alzheimer's disease in elderly institutionalized Canadians. *Annals of Epidemiology*, 14, 319–324.

# 3

# Delirium

## Introduction

Delirium is a common syndrome of acute confusion, with characteristics of rapid onset, an altered level of consciousness, disturbances in attention, orientation, memory, thinking, perception, and behavior, and a fluctuating course (American Psychiatric Association, 1994). Delirium may manifest itself in the patient as hyperactivity, hypoactivity, or as a mixed form of delirium (Sandberg et al., 1999). Signs of delirium include being easily distracted, exhibiting disorganized speech, experiencing periods of altered perception, restlessness, and agitation alternating with lethargy, and showing a clear variability in cognitive function over the course of a day (British Geriatrics Society and Royal College of Physicians, 2006).

A person with dementia has a fivefold increased risk of developing delirium, and approximately three-quarters of patients who develop delirium have already been diagnosed with dementia (Fick et al., 2002, Cole, 2004). Dementia is the major risk factor for the development of delirium in hospitalized older patients (Inouye, 2006). Although delirium is often viewed as a transient state, it can in fact persist for many months and can result in permanent cognitive and functional changes in those who experience it (Marcantonio et al., 2003, Andrew et al., 2005, Fong et al., 2009). Developing delirium increases the risk for older people of poor functional status, dementia, institutionalization, and death (McCusker et al., 2001b, Pitkala et al., 2005, Eeles et al., 2010, Witlox et al., 2010).

## Epidemiology of delirium in dementia

Delirium occurring in a patient with dementia is a common problem. A systematic review of delirium superimposed on dementia in patients across a range of accommodation options found that delirium occurs in between 22 and 89% of people aged 65 and over with dementia (Fick et al., 2002). Lower rates were more likely to be seen in community-dwelling older people, with higher rates observed in residential care.

A retrospective study using a large database from a managed-care organization found that among community-dwelling older people with dementia, 13% had experienced an episode of delirium documented during the 3 years of the study (Fick et al., 2005). A retrospective study of 122 patients in a longitudinal dementia study found that during the 6 years of the study, 25% of the patients had a hospital-confirmed episode of delirium, with almost half of these patients experiencing several episodes of delirium (Baker et al., 1999).

In a prospective study examining an intervention to prevent delirium in hospitalized older people, 32% of the control group of people with dementia developed delirium during their hospitalization (Inouye et al., 1999). A study of 175 older people with dementia undergoing a planned hospital admission showed that 37% of patients developed delirium during their admission (Robertsson et al., 1998). Delirium was more likely to occur in those patients with late-onset Alzheimer's disease (AD), and in the patients with more severe dementia. In an intensive care unit, a prospective cohort study of 118 patients found that patients with dementia were 40% more likely to develop delirium than patients without dementia (McNicoll et al., 2003).

A study of 104 older patients admitted to acute hospital wards from residential-care facilities found that a history of prior cognitive impairment or dementia predicted the occurrence of delirium in hospital. Voyer and colleagues (2006) found that 50% of patients with mild cognitive impairment diagnosed prior to admission developed delirium, compared with 82% of patients with moderate prior cognitive impairment and 86% with severe prior cognitive impairment. In a later cross-sectional study of 155 older people with dementia living in residential-care facilities, Voyer and colleagues found that 70% of these people had a delirium at the time of the study (Voyer et al., 2009).

## Etiology of delirium in dementia

It is suggested that people with dementia are more likely to develop delirium due to an underlying vulnerability in the brain resulting from changes occurring through disease processes such as AD (Inouye and Ferruci, 2006). This predisposes these patients to developing delirium when they undergo surgery, or an acute medical illness occurs, or a medication with anticholinergic effects is prescribed. The existence of this predisposition is supported by findings that indicate that the rate of occurrence of delirium is higher in patients with late-onset AD and vascular dementia, in which there are widespread cortical and subcortical changes, than in patients with earlier-onset AD or frontotemporal dementia, in which changes are predominantly cortical and localized (Robertsson et al., 1999).

There is ongoing debate about the cause and effect relationship between the two conditions, with evidence that delirium may initiate or accelerate an underlying previously undiagnosed dementia (Rockwood et al., 1999, Inouye, 2006). An episode of delirium occurring in a patient with no previous history of dementia, particularly if it occurs after surgery, should always alert clinicians to the possibility of an underlying dementia (Lundstrom et al., 2003).

A number of authors argue that delirium and dementia might simply reflect different stages in the same process because of the clinical, metabolic, and pharmacological similarities (McDonald and Treloar, 1996, Blass and Gibson, 1999, McDonald, 1999). Some risk factors have been shown to be similar for the two conditions. Low educational levels have been noted as a risk factor for the development of dementia (Barnes and Yaffe, 2011), and a secondary analysis of hospital-based studies of delirium has shown that patients with low levels of educational attainment are at increased risk for delirium, compared with older people with higher educational levels (Jones et al., 2006).

Although the pathogenesis of delirium remains poorly understood, there are a number of similarities in underlying disease mechanisms between delirium and dementia, with both conditions associated with cholinergic deficiency and a possible imbalance of the noradrenergic/cholinergic neurotransmitter systems, reduced cerebral oxidative metabolism, disturbances in the sleep/wake cycle, and inflammation (Eikelenboom and Hoogendijk, 1999, Marcantonio et al., 2006). Low brain reserve has been suggested as one of the causes of the cholinergic deficiency (Reyes-Ortiz, 1997), whereas neuroimaging studies have shown decreased cerebral blood flow during a delirium episode compared with blood flow after recovery (Alsop et al., 2006). Other mechanisms postulated in discussions of the pathogenesis of delirium include frontal or parietal cerebral perfusion abnormalities (Fong et al., 2006), disruptions in higher cortical function, as indicated in both neuropsychological testing and neuroimaging studies, and problems in dopaminergic systems as well as cholinergic systems (Mittal et al., 2011).

## Risk factors for delirium in dementia

Although the mechanism is not well understood, it appears that the development of delirium requires a complex interaction between various different factors. These may be either predisposing factors or precipitating factors (Mittal et al., 2011). Dementia is the strongest predisposing factor for the occurrence of delirium, but other factors include age, acute medical illness, the presence of chronic disease, the patient's level of functional autonomy, pain, depression, behavioral disturbances, the number and type of medications taken, dehydration, fever, malnutrition, and anaemia (Joosten et al., 2006, Voyer et al., 2009). In a study of 71 older patients with delirium in an acute hospital setting, predisposing factors associated with moderate to severe delirium were a low Mini-Mental State Examination (MMSE) score, the severity of illness leading to hospitalization, and a low level of functional autonomy, whereas those factors associated with mild delirium were the presence of polypharmacy (particularly narcotics) and a low MMSE score (Voyer et al., 2007).

Precipitating factors for the development of delirium in hospitalized older people include the use of physical restraints, malnutrition, addition of more than three medications during hospitalization, the use of an indwelling bladder catheter, and the occurrence of any iatrogenic event (Inouye and Charpentier, 1996). When looking specifically at people with dementia who develop delirium, precipitating factors have been found to include the use of physical restraints, a low level of sensory stimulation, an inadequate physical environment, and the use of narcotic medications (Voyer et al., 2010).

McCusker and colleagues (2001a) studied likely environmental risk factors for the development of delirium in patients in acute medical wards and found that the number of bed moves or room changes, the absence of a clock or watch, the absence of reading glasses, the absence of a family member, and the presence of physical restraints all increased the severity of delirium in patients both with and without dementia.

## The impact of delirium on dementia

The presence of delirium is associated with an increased length of hospital stay, increased health-service costs, increased mortality, increased rates of admission to residential-care facilities, and increased functional disability (Inouye et al., 1999, McCusker et al., 2003, Saravay et al., 2004, Fick et al., 2005). Symptoms of delirium may persist for up to 6 months following discharge from hospital (Marcantonio et al., 2003), and persistent delirium is a significant predictor of 1-year mortality (Kiely et al., 2009). In a prospective study of patients admitted to a rehabilitation hospital, patients with delirium in combination with dementia were at twice the risk of dying in the following 12 months as patients who had dementia alone, delirium alone, or neither of these conditions (Bellelli et al., 2007).

Delirium occurring in patients with dementia can be a poor prognostic indicator, as delirium has been shown to be a risk factor for mortality, with shorter survival time from dementia onset in those patients who had a documented episode of delirium compared with those who did not (Rockwood et al., 1999, Shigeta and Homma, 2002). In a study of delirium in 441 patients in post-acute care facilities, Yang and colleagues (2009) found that the hypoactive subtype of delirium was associated with the highest risk of mortality at 1 year of follow-up. Because delirium increases the length of hospital stay for any admission (Han et al., 2011), there are then the added increased risks associated with prolonged hospitalization, including falls, pressure areas, hospital-acquired infections, incontinence, and malnutrition (BGS and RCP, 2006).

It may be difficult for clinicians to distinguish the onset of a delirium in a person with dementia, but the consequences of missing the diagnosis of delirium are significant and include early readmission, a longer hospital stay, worsening incontinence, and decreased function (Fick and Foreman, 2000, Andrew et al., 2005). The distinguishing features of delirium include a rapid onset and fluctuating symptoms, compared with a more gradual onset and slowly progressive deterioration of cognition in dementia. However, the significant overlap of symptoms and signs is illustrated in cases of diffuse Lewy body disease (DLBD), in which the signs of fluctuating levels of cognition and visual hallucinations are common to both delirium and dementia (Robinson, 2002, Inouye, 2006).

## Features of delirium in dementia

Although a number of studies have suggested that the clinical features of delirium are similar whether or not a person has dementia (McCusker et al., 2003, Voyer et al., 2006), other studies have reported differences. Edlund and colleagues (2007) studied 717 older people with and without dementia in several settings including an acute general hospital, residential-care facilities, and home settings. They found that those people with dementia who developed delirium were more likely to have had a previous episode of delirium, and were also more likely to be aggressive, agitated, restless, anxious, and poorly oriented, and were more likely to have hallucinations compared with people without dementia who suffered an episode of delirium. They also found that delirium was more common in the evening and at night, and that people with delirium and dementia had greater dependency in activities of daily living (ADL).

Laurila and colleagues (2004) found that the features of clouded consciousness, disorganized thinking and perceptual disturbances were seen more commonly in people with delirium superimposed on dementia, compared with disorientation, motor disturbances, and perceptual disturbances in people with delirium alone. Margiotta and colleagues (2006) found that patients in an acute medical unit who had dementia and developed delirium were more likely to have perceptual disturbances and a fluctuating course than those without dementia who developed delirium. They also found that patients with dementia were vulnerable to delirium at lower levels of medical acuity than those without dementia.

Sandberg and colleagues (1999) conducted a cross-sectional observational study of 315 older people with delirium to examine the prevalence of cognitive, psychiatric, and behavioral symptoms in these patients. Just under half of the study patients had established dementia. Delirium was found to occur at all times of the day and night, with afternoon and evening delirium found to occur more often in those with dementia, and morning delirium occurring more frequently in those without known dementia.

In an observational study of 93 older patients admitted through a hospital emergency department with dementia and the subsequent development of delirium, cognitive symptoms were shown to have appeared before the behavioral symptoms (Saravay et al., 2004), and it was the behavioral disturbances that contributed to the longer length of stay. Also in the hospital setting, the presence of existing cognitive impairment and dementia was found to predict the development of delirium in hip-fracture patients postoperatively (Marcantonio et al., 2001, Kalisvaart et al., 2005).

In a systematic review of reasons for the persistence of delirium, patients with dementia were noted to be more likely to have a prolonged episode of delirium (Dasgupta and Hillier, 2010). The level of prior cognitive impairment influences the severity of the delirium, with longer recovery times and length of hospital stays in those patients with the highest levels of cognitive impairment (Voyer et al., 2006, Voyer et al., 2007, Voyer et al., 2011).

## Assessment and management of delirium in dementia

### Assessment

Delirium is not well recognized, and up to two-thirds of cases of delirium remain undiagnosed (Mittal et al., 2011). In practice it may be very difficult to distinguish delirium from dementia in a patient, so delirium can be missed and symptoms attributed to dementia, particularly in the hypoactive form of delirium (Fick et al., 2002, Edlund et al., 2007). There is also an overlap of cognitive and behavioral symptoms in delirium and dementia – both associated with agitation, aggression, hallucinations, and delusions (Saravay et al., 2004).

The poor recognition of delirium may be due to a lack of knowledge about the condition, difficulty in distinguishing it from dementia, or as is suggested by Rockwood (2002), an ageist attitude toward a condition that requires time and effort to make an accurate diagnosis. The development of delirium in people with existing dementia is even more difficult to identify and less likely to be recognized; thus careful assessment of the person's mental state, with particular attention to any recent changes, is essential (Fick and Foreman, 2000).

A diagnosis of delirium is made using multiple sources of information, including the patient's medical history, physical examination, and behavioral observations, including the use of standardized assessment instruments and gathering information from family and professional carers as to the person's prior level of cognition (Johnson, 2001). The Confusion Assessment Method (CAM) is a widely used and well-validated instrument for the detection of delirium, and it has been used in many hospital-based studies (Inouye et al., 1990). Recently, it has been successfully used to detect delirium in a residential-care environment in a multi-site cohort study of delirium (McCusker et al., 2011), and in a systematic review of bedside instruments to diagnose delirium it was recommended as the instrument of choice (Wong et al., 2010). The National Institute of Clinical Excellence guidance on the management of delirium recommends that a health-care professional who is trained and competent in the diagnosis of delirium should carry out the assessment of delirium, and that if any difficulty arises in distinguishing between the diagnoses of delirium, dementia, and delirium superimposed on dementia, then the delirium should be treated first (Young et al., 2010).

An acute decline in the cognitive function of a person with dementia should suggest the presence of a superimposed episode of delirium. However, these episodes are often not recognized as delirium and may be incorrectly diagnosed as simply a worsening of the dementia (Baker et al., 1999, Fick and Foreman, 2000).

In an attempt to improve the detection of delirium superimposed on dementia in hospitalized patients, a computerized decision support component has been developed and piloted (Fick et al., 2011). A pilot study of its use in 15 hospitalized patients showed that nursing staff were able to successfully use both the assessment and management sections in correctly diagnosing patients.

## Management

There are no specific guidelines for the management of delirium in dementia. However, there are a number of guidelines available with comprehensive evidence-based information to guide the prevention, diagnosis, and management of people with delirium (BGS and RCP, 2006, National Institute for Health and Clinical Excellence, 2010) and it is recommended that these guidelines be used as a basis for management. There have been no trials specifically targeting the management of delirium superimposed on dementia (Fick et al., 2009), although a number of delirium intervention studies have included people with dementia. Much of the following information relates to these studies.

There is conflicting evidence regarding the use of specialized interventions for hospitalized patients with delirium. Although a number of studies have shown that multifactorial and tailored guidelines can improve outcomes for hospitalized patients with delirium or at risk of delirium (Inouye et al., 1999, Marcantonio et al., 2001, Naughton et al., 2005), one large randomized controlled trial of an intervention for patients with delirium failed to show any benefit, and there was no difference in effect between those patients with and without dementia (Cole et al., 2002). Similarly, Marcantonio and colleagues (2001) found their intervention for delirium had no effect on the subgroup of people with dementia. However, a subgroup analysis of the multifactorial delirium prevention trial by Inouye and colleagues (1999) showed that fewer people with dementia in the intervention group (17%) developed delirium than in the control group (32%).

The Cochrane systematic review on the subject of interventions to prevent delirium in hospitalized patients concluded that there was only one trial able to demonstrate any effectiveness of preventive strategies, with consultation by a geriatrician within 24 hours of surgery reducing the incidence of delirium postoperatively (Siddiqi et al., 2007).

The use of a "delirium room" within an acute geriatric ward has been suggested as a way of providing 24-hour intensive nursing care with a multidisciplinary team model of care in a restraint-free environment (Flaherty et al., 2003), and outcomes of an observational study suggest that functional outcomes and length of stay using a delirium room may be similar to those for older patients without delirium (Flaherty et al., 2010). Treating patients with haloperidol as a prophylaxis has been used in an attempt to prevent delirium in older patients undergoing acute or elective hip surgery. The incidence of delirium was not reduced, but there was a decrease in the severity and duration of delirium noted (Kalisvaart et al., 2005). An individualized graduated exercise program delivered to older patients on a medical ward in an acute hospital reduced the incidence of delirium, and there was a trend toward a reduction in the number of falls (Mudge et al., 2008).

Providing rehabilitation treatment in an older person's home rather than in hospital using an outreach model of care has been shown to reduce the chance of delirium occurring (Caplan et al., 2006).

Other interventions include educating staff about delirium, with one study showing that specific education on the detection and management of delirium can increase the recognition of delirium, and improve prevention and management as a result (Tabet et al., 2005). An educational intervention delivered to nursing homes by a delirium practitioner showed positive changes in staff attitudes and practice, and indicates that such an approach is feasible, although incident delirium was not measured (Siddiqi et al., 2011).

It has been suggested that where delirium occurs in a patient with dementia, a focus on supporting attentional skills may assist in recovery from delirium (Kolanowski et al., 2010). A small pilot study of an intervention for the treatment of delirium superimposed on dementia has shown that the implementation of cognitively stimulating activities (such as "Name that tune" and picture puzzles) is feasible, with a trend toward improvement over time in the intervention group (Kolanowski et al., 2011).

The pharmacological management of delirium should be targeted toward the underlying causes, such as treating with antibiotics for infection, and with analgesics for pain relief. If the patient is experiencing behavioral or psychological symptoms that are causing distress, such as agitation, aggression, hallucinations, or delusions, antipsychotic medication may be appropriate. The Cochrane systematic review on the use of antipsychotics in delirium concludes that there is evidence for the use of haloperidol, risperidone, and olanzapine (Lonergan et al., 2007). The Cochrane review of the use of benzodiazepines in delirium concluded that there is no evidence for their use except in alcohol-withdrawal-related delirium (Lonergan et al., 2009).

Melatonin has been used successfully to treat sundowning and agitated behaviors in older people with dementia (de Jonghe et al., 2010), and the authors suggest that as similar disturbances related to the sleep/wake cycle are also seen in delirium, melatonin might have a similar positive effect on delirium. There has been one randomized controlled trial of delirium prevention reported using a physiological dose of melatonin (0.5 mg daily) in older people, some of whom had dementia. Melatonin or placebo was given to 145 older patients on admission to an acute hospital ward for the following 14 days or until discharge. Approximately 20% of these patients had a confirmed dementia. There was a 15.6% decrease in the absolute risk of delirium in the melatonin-treated group compared with the placebo group, and melatonin was well tolerated. There was no difference in the severity of delirium or hospital length of stay (Al-Aama et al., 2011).

## Recommendations

1. Expect delirium in unwell and hospitalized older patients with dementia and use a simple screening test such as the CAM regularly to detect delirium. Look for a patient who is easily distracted, has periods of altered perception, exhibits

disorganized speech, has periods of both restlessness with agitation and lethargy, and who has a clear variation in cognitive function over the course of a day.

2. Find the cause of the delirium and treat symptomatically. This includes correcting fluid and electrolyte imbalances, treating infection, ceasing inappropriate medication (particularly medications with anticholinergic effects), considering alcohol or benzodiazepine withdrawal, and managing hypoxia.

3. Nurse in an appropriately specialized ward environment (e.g., a delirium room) and ensure that spectacles and hearing aids are available, and the patient has a clock or watch available to assist in orientation. The patient should be kept as mobile as possible.

4. Avoid the use of restraints, and keep use of sedative or antipsychotic medications to a minimum. If constant supervision is required, consider encouraging family members to be present or arrange the use of one-to-one nursing.

5. Discourage patient bed moves and changes in location.

---

**Case studies**

Mrs. C is a 79-year-old woman with moderate dementia, cared for by her husband and daughter at home with assistance from community nurses. Mrs. C fell in her bathroom and sustained a fractured hip, requiring hospitalization and surgery. She was confused on admission, and following surgical fixation of her fracture she became even more confused, and was agitated and experiencing visual hallucinations. She was transferred to a dedicated delirium management ward, where she was given regular analgesia, kept well hydrated through checking of her electrolytes and urine output, and her family were encouraged to sit with her, particularly in the afternoon and evening. She was mobilized in a walking frame on the day after surgery and her urinary catheter was removed. Mrs. C became much less agitated and confused over the subsequent days and her husband said that she was almost back to normal. She was transferred to the rehabilitation ward a week postoperatively to continue mobilization.

Mr. D is an 81-year-old man who lives with his son in his own home. He has a long past history of chronic airflow limitation (CAL) and has had several hospital admissions with an acute exacerbation of his CAL during which he subsequently developed delirium. He became confused, aggressive, and difficult to manage in this condition, and required individual one-to-one nursing, sedation, and assistance from family members. After discharge from his fourth admission he was investigated for cognitive impairment, and was found to have an early dementia, probably a mixed vascular and Alzheimer's dementia. He was commenced on a cholinesterase inhibitor with modest improvement on cognitive testing. Mr. D's subsequent admissions to hospital with exacerbation of CAL became easier to manage, as nursing staff were aware of his dementia and he was nursed in an appropriate environment. He was much less confused and required a shorter length of time in hospital. He has remained cognitively stable for more than 12 months.

---

**Key points**

- Dementia is the strongest risk factor for the occurrence of delirium, and people with dementia have a fivefold increased risk of developing delirium compared with people without dementia.
- Two-thirds of cases of delirium occur in people with dementia, but many cases go unrecognized, as dementia is blamed for the symptoms.
- Lower educational level and greater severity of dementia predict greater severity of delirium.
- There are likely to be similar underlying mechanisms for dementia and delirium, including decreased cerebral metabolism, cholinergic deficits, and inflammation.

## References

Al-Aama, T., Brymer, C., Gutmanis, I., et al. (2011). Melatonin decreases delirium in elderly patients: a randomized, placebo-controlled trial. *International Journal of Geriatric Psychiatry*, 26, 687–694.

Alsop, D., Fearing, M., Johnson, K., et al. (2006). The role of neuroimaging in elucidating delirium pathophysiology. *Journal of Gerontology: Medical Sciences*, 61A, 1287–1293.

American Psychiatric Association. (1994). Delirium, dementia, and amnestic and other cognitive disorders. In: *Diagnostic and statistical manual of mental disorders*. 4th edn. Washington DC: American Psychiatric Association.

Andrew, M., Freter, S., Rockwood, K. (2005). Incomplete functional recovery after delirium in elderly people: a prospective cohort study. *BMC Geriatrics*, 5, 5.

Baker, F., Wiley, C., Kokmen, E., et al. (1999). Delirium episodes during the course of clinically diagnosed Alzheimer's disease. *Journal of the National Medical Association*, 91, 625–630.

Barnes, D. and Yaffe, K. (2011). The projected effect of risk factor reduction on Alzheimer's disease prevalence. *Lancet Neurology*, 10, 819–828.

Bellelli, G., Frisoni, G., Turco, R., et al. (2007). Delirium superimposed on dementia predicts 12-month survival in elderly patients discharged from a post acute rehabilitation facility. *Journals of Gerontology: Medical Sciences*, 62, 1306–1309.

Blass, J. and Gibson, G. (1999). Cerebrometabolic aspects of delirium in relationship to dementia. *Dementia and Geriatric Cognitive Disorders*, 10, 335–338.

British Geriatrics Society and Royal College of Physicians. *Guidelines for the prevention, diagnosis and management of delirium in older people*. Concise guidance to good clinical practice series, No 6. London: RCP, 2006.

Caplan, G., Coconis, J., Board, N., et al. (2006). Does home treatment affect delirium : a randomised controlled trial of rehabilitation of elderly and care at home or usual treatment (the REACH-OUT trial). *Age and Ageing*, 35, 53–60.

Cole, M. (2004). Delirium in elderly patients. *The American Journal of Geriatric Psychiatry*, 12, 7–21.

Cole, M., McCusker, J., Bellavance, F., et al. (2002) Systematic detection and multi-disciplinary care of delirium in older medical patients: a randomized trial. *Canadian Medical Association Journal*, 167, 753–759.

Dasgupta, M. and Hillier, L. (2010). Factors associated with prolonged delirium: a systematic review. *International Psychogeriatrics*, 22, 373–394.

De Jonghe, A., Korevaar, J., van Munster, B., et al. (2010). Effectiveness of mela-tonin treatment on circadian rhythm disturbances in dementia. Are there impli-cations for delirium? A systematic review. *International Journal of Geriatric Psychiatry*, 25, 1201–1208.

Edlund, A., Lundstrom, M., Sandberg, O., et al. (2007). Symptom profile of delir-ium in older people with and without dementia. *Journal of Geriatric Psychiatry & Neurology*, 20, 166–171.

Eeles, E., Hubbard, R., White, S., et al. (2010). Hospital use, institutionalization and mortality associated with delirium. *Age & Ageing*, 39, 470–475.

Eikelenboom, P. and Hoogendijk, W. (1999). Do delirium and Alzheimer's demen-tia share specific pathogenetic mechanisms? *Dementia and Geriatric Cognitive Disorders*, 10, 319–324.

Fick, D., Agostini, J., Inouye, S. (2002). Delirium superimposed on dementia: a systematic review. *Journal of the American Geriatrics Society*, 50, 1723–1732.

Fick, D. and Foreman, M. (2000). Consequences of not recognizing delirium superimposed on dementia in hospitalized elderly individuals. *Journal of Gerontological Nursing*, 26, 30–40.

Fick, D., Kolanowski, A., Beattie, E., et al. (2009). Delirium in early-stage Alzheimer's disease: enhancing cognitive reserve as a possible preventive meas-ure. *Journal of Gerontological Nursing*, 35, 30–43.

Fick, D., Kolanowski, A., Waller, J., et al. (2005). Delirium superimposed on dementia in a community dwelling managed care population: a 3 year retro-spective study of occurrence, costs and utilisation. *Journals of Gerontology: Medical Sciences*, 60A, 748–753.

Fick, D., Steis, M., Mion, L., et al. (2011) Computerized decision support for delirium superimposed on dementia in older adults. *Journal of Gerontological Nursing*, 37, 39–47.

Flaherty, J., Steele, K., Chibnall, J., et al. (2010). An ACE Unit with a Delirium Room may improve function and equalize length of stay among older deli-rious medical inpatients. *Journal of Gerontology: Medical Sciences*, 65A, 1387–1392.

Flaherty, J., Tariq, S., Raghavan, S., et al. (2003) A model for managing delirious older inpatients. *Journal of the American Geriatrics Society*, 51, 1031–1035.

Fong, T., Bogardus, S., Daftary, A., et al. (2006). Cerebral perfusion changes in older delirious patients using 99mTc HMPAO SPECT. *Journal of Gerontology: Medical Sciences*, 61A, 1294–1299.

Fong, T., Jones, R., Shi, P., et al. (2009) Delirium accelerates cognitive decline in Alzheimer disease. *Neurology*, 72, 1570–1575.

Han, J., Eden, S., Shintani, A., et al. (2011). Delirium in older Emergency Department patients is an independent predictor of hospital length of stay. *Academic Emergency Medicine*, 18, 451–457.

Inouye, S. (2006). Delirium in older persons. *New England Journal of Medicine*, 354, 1157–1165.

Inouye, S., Bogardus, S., Charpentier, P., et al. (1999). A multicomponent intervention to prevent delirium in hospitalized older patients. *New England Journal of Medicine*, 340, 669–676.

Inouye, S. and Charpentier, P. (1996). Precipitating factors for delirium in hospitalized elderly persons. Predictive model and interrelationship with baseline vulnerability. *Journal of the American Medical Association*, 275, 852–857.

Inouye, S. and Ferruci, L. (2006). Elucidating the pathophysiology of delirium and the interrelationship of delirium and dementia. *Journal of Gerontology: Medical Sciences*, 61A, 1277–1280.

Inouye, S., VanDyck, C., Alessi, C., et al. (1990) Clarifying confusion: the Confusion Assessment Method: a new method for detection of delirium. *Annals of Internal Medicine*, 113, 941–948.

Johnson, M. (2001). Assessing confused patients. *Journal of Neurology, Neurosurgery & Neuropsychiatry*, 71, 7–12.

Jones, R., Yang, F., Zhang, Y., et al. (2006). Does educational attainment contribute to risk for delirium? A potential role for cognitive reserve. *Journal of Gerontology: Medical Sciences*, 61A, 1307–1311.

Joosten, E., Lemiengre, J., Nelis, T., et al. (2006). Is anaemia a risk factor for delirium in an acute geriatric population? *Gerontology*, 52, 382–385.

Kalisvaart, K., de Jonghe, J., Bogaards, M., et al. (2005). Haloperidol prophylaxis for elderly hip-surgery patients at risk for delirium: a randomized placebo-controlled study. *Journal of the American Geriatrics Society*, 53, 1658–1666.

Kiely, D., Marcantonio, E., Inouye, S., et al. (2009). Persistent delirium predicts greater mortality. *Journal of the American Geriatrics Society*, 57, 55–61.

Kolanowski, A., Fick, D., Clare, L., et al. (2010). An intervention for delirium superimposed on dementia based on cognitive reserve theory. *Aging & Mental Health*, 14, 232–242.

Kolanowksi, A., Fick, D., Clare, L., et al. (2011). Pilot study of a nonpharmacological intervention for delirium superimposed on dementia. *Research in Gerontological Nursing*, 4, 161–167.

Laurila, J., Pitkala, K., Strandberg, T., et al. (2004). Delirium among patients with and without dementia: does the diagnosis according to DSM-IV differ from the previous classifications? *International Journal of Geriatric Psychiatry*, 19, 271–277.

Lonergan, E., Britton, A., Luxenberg, J. (2007). Antipsychotics for delirium. *Cochrane Database of Systematic Reviews*, 2, CD 005594.

Lonergan, E., Luxenberg, J., Areosa Sastre, A. (2009). Benzodiazepines for delirium. *Cochrane Database of Systematic Reviews*, 4, CD006379.

Lundstrom, M., Edlund, A., Bucht, G., et al. (2003). Dementia after delirium in patients with femoral neck fractures. *Journal of the American Geriatrics Society*, 51, 1002–1006.

Marcantonio, E., Flacker, J., Wright, R., et al. (2001). Reducing delirium after hip fracture: a randomized trial. *Journal of the American Geriatrics Society*, 49, 516–522.

Marcantonio, E., Rudolph, J., Culley, D., et al. (2006). Serum biomarkers for delirium. *Journals of Gerontology: Medical Sciences*, 61A, 1281–1286.

Marcantonio, E., Simon, S., Bergmann, M., et al. (2003). Delirium symptoms in post-acute care: prevalent, persistent, and associated with poor functional recovery. *Journal of the American Geriatrics Society*, 51, 4–9.

Margiotta, A., Bianchetti, A., Ranieri, P., et al. (2006). Clinical characteristics and risk factors of delirium in demented and not demented elderly medical inpatients. *Journal of Nutrition, Health & Aging*, 10, 535–539.

McCusker, J., Cole, M., Abrahamowicz, M., et al. (2001a) Environmental risk factors for delirium in hospitalized older people. *Journal of the American Geriatrics Society*, 49, 1327–1334.

McCusker, J., Cole, M., Dendukuri, N., et al. (2001b). Delirium in older medical inpatients and subsequent cognitive and functional status: a prospective study. *Canadian Medical Association Journal*, 165, 575–583.

McCusker, J., Cole, M., Dendukuri, N., et al. (2003). The course of delirium in older medical outpatients: a prospective study. *Journal of General Internal Medicine*, 18, 696–704.

McCusker, J., Cole, M., Voyer, P., et al. (2011). Use of nurse-observed symptoms of delirium in long-term care: effects on prevalence and outcomes of delirium. *International Psychogeriatrics*, 23, 602–608.

McDonald, A. (1999). Can delirium be separated from dementia? *Dementia and Geriatric Cognitive Disorders*, 10, 386–388.

McDonald, A. and Treloar, A. (1996). Delirium and dementia; are they distinct? *Journal of the American Geriatrics Society*, 44, 1001–1002.

McNicoll, L., Pisani, M., Ahang, Y., et al. (2003). Delirium in the Intensive Care Unit: occurrence and clinical course in older patients. *Journal of the American Geriatrics Society*, 51, 591–598.

Mittal, V., Muralee, S., Williamson, D., et al. (2011). Delirium in the elderly: a comprehensive review. *American Journal of Alzheimer's Disease & Other Dementias*, 26, 97–109.

Mudge, A., Giebel, A., Cutler, A. (2008). Exercising body and mind: an integrated approach to functional independence in hospitalized older people. *Journal of the American Geriatrics Society*, 56, 630–635.

National Institute for Health and Clinical Excellence. (2010). Delirium: diagnosis, prevention and management. (Clinical guideline 103). Available at: http://www.nice.org.uk/CG103 [Accessed February 14, 2012].

Naughton, B., Saltzman, S., Ramadan, F., et al. (2005). A multifactorial intervention to reduce prevalence of delirium and shorten hospital length of stay. *Journal of the American Geriatrics Society*, 53, 18–23.

Pitkala, K., Laurila, J., Strandberg, T., et al. (2005). Prognostic significance of delirium in frail older people. *Dementia and Geriatric Cognitive Disorders*, 19, 158–163.

Reyes-Ortiz, C. (1997). Delirium, dementia and brain reserve. *Journal of the American Geriatrics Society*, 45, 778–779.

Robertsson, B., Blennow, K., Gottfries, C., et al. (1998). Delirium in dementia. *International Journal of Geriatric Psychiatry*, 13, 49–56.

Robertsson, B., Olsson, L., Wallin, A. (1999). Occurrence of delirium in different regional brain syndromes. *Dementia and Geriatric Cognitive Disorders*, 10, 278–283.

Robinson, M. (2002). Probably Lewy body dementia presenting as "delirium." *Psychosomatics*, 43, 84–86.

Rockwood, K. (2002). Out of the furrow and into the fire: where do we go with delirium? *Canadian Medical Association Journal*, 167, 763–764.

Rockwood, K., Cosway, S., Carver, D., et al. (1999). The risk of dementia and death after delirium. *Age & Ageing*, 28, 551–556.

Sandberg, O., Gustafson, Y., Brannstrom, B., et al. (1999). Clinical profile of delirium in older patients. *Journal of the American Geriatrics Society*, 47, 1300–1306.

Saravay, S., Kaplowitz, M., Kurek, J., et al. (2004). How do delirium and dementia increase length of stay of elderly general medical inpatients? *Psychosomatics*, 45, 235–242.

Shigeta, M. and Homma, A. (2002). Survival and risk factors for mortality in elderly patients with dementia. *Current Opinions in Psychiatry*, 15, 423–426.

Siddiqi, N., Holt, R., Britton, A., et al. (2007). Interventions for preventing delirium in hospitalized patients. *Cochrane Database of Systematic Reviews*, 2, CD005563.

Siddiqi, J., Young, J., House, A., et al. (2011). Stop Delirium! A complex intervention to prevent delirium in care homes: a mixed-methods feasibility study. *Age & Ageing*, 40, 90–98.

Tabet, N., Hudson, S., Sweeney, V., et al. (2005). An educational intervention can prevent delirium on acute medical wards. *Age & Ageing*, 34, 152–156.

Voyer, P., Cole, M., McCusker, J., et al. (2006). Prevalence and symptoms of delirium superimposed on dementia. *Clinical Nursing Research*, 15, 46–66.

Voyer, P., McCusker, J., Cole, M., et al. (2007). Factors associated with delirium severity among older patients. *Journal of Clinical Nursing*, 16, 819–831.

Voyer, P., Richard, S., Doucet, L., et al. (2009). Predisposing factors associated with delirium among demented long-term care residents. *Clinical Nursing Research*, 18, 153–171.

Voyer, P., Richard, S., Doucet, L., et al. (2010) Examination of the multifactorial model of delirium among long-term care residents with dementia. *Geriatric Nursing*, 31, 105–114.

Voyer, P., Richard, S., Doucet, L., et al. (2011). Factors associated with delirium severity among older persons with dementia. *Journal of Neuroscience Nursing*, 43, 62–69.

Witlox, J., Eurelings, L., de Jonghe, J., et al. (2010) Delirium in elderly patients and the risk of postdischarge mortality, institutionalization and dementia. *Journal of the American Medical Association*, 304, 443–451.

Wong, C., Holroyd-Leduc, J., Simel, D., et al. (2010). Does this patient have delirium?: value of bedside instruments. *Journal of the American Medical Association*, 304, 779–786.

Yang, F., Marcantonio, E., Inouye, S., et al. (2009). Phenomenological subtypes of delirium in older persons: patterns, prevalence, and prognosis. *Psychosomatics*, 50, 248–254.

Young, J., Murthy, L., Westby, M., et al. on behalf of the Guideline Development Group. (2010). Diagnosis, prevention, and management of delirium: summary of NICE guidance. *British Medical Journal*, 341, 247–249.

# 4

# Epilepsy

## Introduction

Epileptic seizures are defined as brief, unprovoked disturbances of consciousness, behavior, motor function, or sensation (McAreavey et al., 1992), and they are known to occur more frequently in older people (Hauser, 1992, Forsgren et al., 1996, Pugh et al., 2009). However, the likelihood of seizures in people with dementia is further increased compared with an age-matched population (Amatniek et al., 2006), and it has been suggested that many of these, particularly partial seizures, are not detected and remain undiagnosed (Mendez and Lim, 2003).

Although seizures were not one of the clinical features described by Alois Alzheimer in his early case reports, they were mentioned as a feature of Alzheimer's disease (AD) in a 1936 description of a 53-year-old patient with neuropathologically confirmed disease (Hannah, 1936). It is now evident that AD, along with other dementias, is associated with an increased risk of developing epileptic seizures. The clinical diagnostic criteria for AD outlined by the National Institute of Neurological and Communicative Disorders and Stroke/Alzheimer's Disease and Related Disorders Association (NINCDS–ADRDA) Work Group now include seizures as a clinical feature consistent with a diagnosis of Alzheimer's disease (McKhann et al., 1984).

## Epidemiology and prevalence of seizures in dementia

A large number of studies have confirmed that people with dementia have a significantly higher chance of developing new-onset seizures during the course of their disease than those without dementia. Many of these studies have looked specifically at people with AD and have reported results indicating that seizures may occur in up to 23% of people with the disease (Mendez and Lim, 2003). A study by

Hauser et al. (1986) of 81 patients with AD found that 10% of these patients had suffered a seizure, which demonstrates a 10-fold increase in seizure risk compared with the older population without dementia. In a group of 87 older male patients in residential care, Rudman and colleagues (1988) found that 18% had suffered at least one seizure, and "organic brain disease" (including AD) was considered the reason. In a prospective study of 44 patients with AD, seven (16%) developed seizures in the later stages of the disease (Romanelli et al., 1990). A review of 208 patients with dementia in institutional care by McAreavey et al. (1992) found that 9% had suffered at least two seizures. In a clinicopathological study of 446 patients with AD (confirmed at autopsy), Mendez and colleagues found that 17% of these patients had suffered at least one seizure (Mendez et al., 1994).

Volicer and colleagues (1995) studied 75 patients with severe AD and found that 21% developed seizures during the course of their disease. Some deterioration in language and function was noted in a number of these patients following the seizures. Hesdorffer and colleagues (1996) reviewed 285 patients with seizures. They found that the presence of diagnosed AD increased the risk of developing new-onset seizures sixfold, and the presence of other types of dementia (particularly vascular dementia) increased the risk by a factor of eight. In a cohort study of 236 patients recruited following a diagnosis of AD, 7% of these patients developed seizures during the follow-up period (Amatniek et al., 2006). The authors noted that the diagnosis of AD increased the risk of having seizures in patients aged 50–59 years by a factor of 87, compared with the non-AD population.

In contrast to these studies, another prospective cohort study of 453 patients with probable AD found that only 1.5% of these patients experienced seizures (Scarmeas et al., 2009). The seizures were mainly generalized convulsions and were diagnosed using detailed case reviews by medical practitioners experienced in epilepsy. Although the seizure incidence in this study was low, this result still showed an eightfold increase in the risk of unprovoked seizures compared with the general population. Rao and colleagues (2009) performed a retrospective review of 1738 case records of patients in an Alzheimer's disease patient registry, finding that 3.6% of patients with dementia had documented seizure activity, mainly consisting of complex partial seizures. The authors also noted that 80% of patients with seizures had an excellent response to antiepileptic therapy.

Examining seizures from a different perspective, in a large study of veterans over the age of 66 years researchers investigated risk factors for new-onset seizures (Pugh et al., 2009). They found that patients with cerebrovascular disease as well as dementia had a fourfold increased risk of developing new-onset seizures compared with a control group of older patients without seizures. In a prospective study of 160 older people who had suffered a seizure, dementia was diagnosed in 18% of patients, and AD was considered to be the cause in 7% of these patients (Forsgren et al., 1996).

Although many studies have examined seizures in people with AD, other dementias are also recognized as a cause of seizures. The presence of vascular disease in the brain increases the chance of seizures occurring, and a prospective study of 202 stroke patients showed that those with preexisting dementia had a fourfold increased chance of developing seizures following a stroke, compared with patients without a known dementia (Cordonnier et al., 2005). A review of 100 neuropathologically confirmed cases of AD, AD with Lewy bodies (AD+LB) (both AD changes and Lewy bodies present), and diffuse Lewy body dementia (DLBD) indicated that seizures are likely to occur more commonly in DLBD than in AD, and the seizures are likely to occur earlier in the course of the disease (Weiner et al., 2003).

In patients with Huntington's disease, seizures feature early after disease onset, and are more commonly seen in patients who develop the disease at a younger age (Brackenridge, 1980). In Creutzfeldt–Jakob disease (CJD), in which rapidly progressive dementia and myoclonus are typical symptoms, seizures occur in 10–15% of patients (Neufeld et al., 2003, Wieser et al., 2006). A number of cases have also been reported of both convulsive and nonconvulsive status epilepticus presenting as a symptom of the disease (Cohen et al., 2004, Fernandez-Torre et al., 2004).

In people with Down syndrome, in whom the neuropathological changes of AD are seen in the brain from as early as the third decade of life, seizures are reported to be common, and to be increasingly common as the person with Down syndrome ages. A cross-sectional study of 191 adults with Down syndrome indicated that approximately 10% overall suffered seizures, with almost 50% of those over the age of 50 years having had at least one documented seizure, usually associated with a diagnosis of dementia (McVicker et al., 1994). In a small study of 15 cases of patients with Down syndrome, more than half were found to be having seizures, and these were often associated with the onset of dementia symptoms (Lott and Lai, 1982). In a larger study of 351 patients with Down syndrome, 10% of the individuals studied had a history of seizures, and in those patients over 60 years of age, 31% had some seizure history (Collacott, 1993). Similarly, Johannsen et al. (1996) found a 13% overall prevalence of seizures in a study of 85 people with Down syndrome, which rose to 24% in those over the age of 50 years. Several of these authors have suggested that these findings indicate that seizures might be a manifestation of the dementia process.

## Epilepsy as a risk factor for dementia

Although early studies commented that epilepsy and frequent seizures did not appear to be implicated as a risk factor in developing dementia (Brackenridge, 1980), more recent epidemiological studies have suggested that epilepsy may present a mild risk factor for later developing dementia. Examining three national morbidity registers, Breteler and colleagues (1995) found that patients with epilepsy appeared to have a 1.5 times increased risk of developing dementia compared with a reference group. They also postulated that epilepsy might be an initial manifestation of AD changes in the brain. Gaitatzis and colleagues (2004) extracted data from a national general practice research database and found that neurodegenerative conditions, including AD and other dementias, appeared more frequently in people with epilepsy than in those without epilepsy.

Motamedi and Meador (2003), Ortinski and Meador (2004), Martin et al. (2005) and Brown (2006) have suggested that the intellectual deterioration often seen in epilepsy might be due to other factors, including the direct effect of seizures on the brain or the influence of antiepileptic drugs. This latter factor was investigated in a large national cohort study that found that older people who were taking antiepileptic drugs were at a higher risk of developing dementia compared with those not taking these drugs (Carter et al., 2007). However, this study did not find that epilepsy itself was associated with an increased risk of developing AD or dementia. In a review of cognitive and brain aging in patients with chronic epilepsy, Hermann and colleagues (2008) concluded that cognitive changes often occur in chronic epilepsy and noted that these may be related to upregulated amyloid precursor protein and increased rates of amyloid plaque deposition. They also highlighted the overrepresentation of known dementia risk factors in people with epilepsy, including vascular, inflammatory, and lifestyle factors.

## Etiology of seizures

The pathogenesis of seizures in dementia remains unclear and a number of theories have been proposed. One possible cause is thought to be the development of epileptogenic lesions associated with the selective loss of neurones and glial cells in the parietal, neocortical, and hippocampal areas (Forstl et al., 1992, Mendez and Lim, 2003). Occult vascular lesions have been suggested as another possible source of seizures, as have alterations in neurotransmitters, particularly acetylcholine and dopamine (Larner, 2010). Axonal sprouting, which occurs in the brain with AD, may result in the formation of aberrant connections between neurones, which have been put forward as a possible cause for seizures (Lozsadi and Larner, 2006). Noebels (2011) has suggested that the combination of synaptic hyperactivity due to a loss of inhibitory mechanisms in AD, together with elevated levels of amyloid protein, can lead to the occurrence of seizures. The involvement of amyloid overexpression in seizure etiology is supported by the common occurrence of epilepsy in familial AD, with mutations in the genes encoding amyloid precursor protein (Palop and Mucke, 2009), and amyloid cleaving enzymes (Velez-Pardo et al., 2004).

Although stroke and cerebrovascular disease are known causes of seizures, the presence of other disease in the brain does not appear to increase the chance of seizures occurring. Where comparisons have been made between AD patients with and without seizures, no apparent distinction can be made between these groups with respect to the presence of hypertension, diabetes, or other medical illnesses, the use of psychotropic drugs or other medication, or alcohol use (Mendez and Lim, 2003). There are a number of medications used in the treatment of dementia that may potentially lower the seizure threshold. These include the antipsychotics and the cholinesterase inhibitors (Mendez and Lim, 2003). Although this possibility should be considered, there is currently little evidence that these medications do increase the occurrence of seizures in people with dementia.

## Features of seizures in dementia

Despite the fact seizures may occur at any stage in the course of dementia, a number of studies report that seizures mostly tend to occur later in the disease process, typically occurring 6–7 years after dementia is diagnosed (Romanelli et al., 1990, Forstl et al., 1992, Volicer et al., 1995). Although seizures are more likely to occur later in the disease process, they have also been noted earlier in AD in some individuals, with a number of patients in a memory clinic cohort study exhibiting seizure activity around the time of diagnosis (Lozsadi and Larner, 2006). Conversely, other studies have not shown any association between disease duration or cognitive performance and the presence of seizures (Scarmeas et al., 2009).

The risk for developing seizures appears to be much higher in younger AD patients (those under the age of 65 years) than in older patients, with studies reporting up to an 87-fold increase in the risk of seizures among the younger age group (Mendez et al., 1994, Amatniek et al., 2006).

Seizures in dementia are usually partial in nature (Larner, 2010), although generalized onset seizures are also seen (Hesdorffer et al., 1996). Complex partial seizures were the seizure type experienced most commonly, as shown in a retrospective review of 63 patients with epilepsy (Rao et al., 2009).

## Management of seizures in dementia

Diagnosis of seizures in people with dementia can be problematic owing to difficulties associated with history-taking and examination, and the concurrent presence of other conditions such as syncope or transient ischemic attacks. In addition to taking a thorough clinical history with confirmatory information from family or carers as an essential first step, a detailed physical and neurological examination should also be performed. Symptoms and signs of seizures may be subtle, and complex partial seizures may go unrecognized given that their characteristics may mimic dementia symptoms, such as transient amnesia or wandering (Rabinowicz et al., 2000). Seizures may also present as a fall or syncope with consequences involving a head injury and subdural haematoma, or a hip or other fracture (Blume, 2003).

It is important to exclude other potential causes of seizures such as traumatic brain injury, tumor, stroke, metabolic disturbance, or infection (Caramelli and Castro, 2005). Routine laboratory investigations and neuroimaging may be appropriate in these patients to exclude other potentially treatable seizure causes. Unless taken during a seizure, an electroencephalogram is rarely diagnostic, and may just show a general slowing (Mendez and Lim, 2003).

Treatment of seizures is important in patients with AD, and it is recommended that therapy be instituted after two seizures, given the high risk of further seizures occurring (Hauser et al., 1998). There have been no specific trials addressing drug treatment of seizures in dementia, so information from drug trials in epilepsy in the general population has been extrapolated for these patients. In a retrospective study of patients with dementia and epilepsy by Rao and colleagues (2009), the authors noted that the majority of patients had a very good response to antiepileptic therapy. However, about one-third of patients experienced adverse events, which included confusion, mental slowing, drowsiness, ataxia, and visual disturbances. It is important to remember that pharmacokinetic and pharmaco-dynamic changes occur with aging, and care needs to be taken in prescribing these drugs, with slow titration and regular monitoring of blood levels recommended (Caramelli and Castro, 2005). The possible interactions with concurrent medications such as antipsychotics, antidepressants, and the cholinesterase inhibitors also need to be considered.

Mendez and Lim (2003) suggest starting with low doses of carbamazepine (100 mg/day), valproic acid (125 mg/day), gabapentin (300 mg/day), or lamotrigine (25 mg/day) as first-line monotherapy for seizures in older patients with dementia. These dosages can be gradually titrated upward. Levetiracetam has also been used in an open-label prospective study of 25 patients with AD and seizures, with the authors of that study reporting that 72% of the patients were free from seizures for at least 1 year on 1000–1500 mg/day (Belcastro et al., 2007).

## Recommendations

1. Consider the possibility of seizures if people with dementia or their carers report the occurrence of falls, syncope or faints, altered mental status, or acute confusional episodes.
2. Be aware that seizures may be atypical and the EEG may not be conclusive.
3. If seizures are suspected, exclude other possible causes for new-onset seizures.
4. If two or more seizures have occurred, consider treatment with anticonvulsants such as carbamazepine, valproic acid, gabapentin, or lamotrigine.

---

### Case studies

Mrs. A is an 83-year-old woman who lives in supported accommodation. She has moderate AD and requires some assistance with personal care but is otherwise independent. She enjoys outings on the facility bus and walking in the garden. Over the course of a few months, she had several unexplained falls, during which she was found on the ground with no memory of the fall. One of the falls resulted in a fractured wrist, and staff were reluctant to allow her outside without supervision. She also fell in her room and fractured her shoulder, subsequently requiring hospital admission. Mrs. A was investigated for a possible cause for her falls, with no obvious cause found. During her time in hospital she was observed to suddenly lose consciousness and fall while walking to the dining room. A seizure was considered to be the cause, and an electroencephalogram was arranged for later that day. It was not diagnostic of epilepsy, but Mrs. A was commenced on valproic acid on the basis of her history of unexplained falls. She has had no more falls during 18 months of follow-up.

Mr. B is a 61-year-old man who lives at home with his wife. He has early Alzheimer's disease. His wife described a number of periods of confusion lasting several minutes during which Mr. B did not recognize his family members or friends, and could not remember where he was or what he had been doing. He recovered after about 15 minutes and had no memory of the episodes. He was fully investigated with MRI imaging and EEG with no obvious cause. Seizures were considered the most likely cause and he was commenced on carbamazepine. He was initially quite sleepy on this and was changed to lamotrigine. Over the past 9 months he has had no further episodes of amnesia.

---

**Key points**

- People with dementia have a sixfold increased risk of having a seizure compared with the normal population.
- Between 5 and 10% of people with dementia are likely to have a seizure.
- Seizures are more likely to occur in younger people with Alzheimer's disease than in older people, and seizure incidence is higher in patients with vascular dementia than in those with Alzheimer's disease.

## References

Amatniek, J., Hauser, W., Delcastillo-Castaneda, C., et al. (2006). Incidence and predictors of seizures in patients with Alzheimer's disease. *Epilepsia*, 47, 867–872.

Belcastro, V., Costa, C., Galletti, F., et al. (2007). Levetiracetam monotherapy in Alzheimer patients with late-onset seizures: a prospective observational study. *European Journal of Neurology*, 14, 1176–1178.

Blume, W. (2003). Diagnosis and management of epilepsy. *Canadian Medical Association Journal*, 168, 441–448.

Brackenridge, C.J. (1980). Factors influencing dementia and epilepsy in Huntington's disease of early onset. *Acta Neurologica Scandinavia*, 62, 305–311.

Breteler, M., de Groot, R.R.M., van Romunde L.K.J., et al. (1995). Risk of dementia in patients with Parkinson's disease, epilepsy, and severe head trauma: a register-based follow-up study. *American Journal of Epidemiology*, 142, 1300–1305.

Brown, S. (2006). Deterioration. *Epilepsia*, 47, 19–23.

Caramelli, P. and Castro, L.H.M. (2005). Dementia associated with epilepsy. *International Psychogeriatrics*, 17, S195–S206.

Carter, M.D., Weaver, D.F., Joudrey, H.R., et al. (2007). Epilepsy and antiepileptic drug use in elderly people as risk factors for dementia. *Journal of the Neurological Sciences*, 252, 169–172.

Cohen, D., Kutluay, E., Edwards, J., et al. (2004) Sporadic Creutzfeldt-Jakob disease presenting with nonconvulsive status epilepticus. *Epilepsy & Behaviour*, 5, 792–796.

Collacott, R.A. (1993). Epilepsy, dementia and adaptive behaviour in Down Syndrome. *Journal of Intellectual Disability Research*, 37, 153–160.

Cordonnier, C., Henon, H., Derambure P., et al. (2005). Influence of pre-existing dementia on the risk of post-stroke epileptic seizures. *Journal of Neurology, Neurosurgery and Psychiatry*, 76, 1649–1653.

Fernandez-Torre, J.L., Solar, D.M., Astudillo, A., et al. (2004). Creutzfeldt-Jakob disease and nonconvulsive status epilepticus. *Clinical Neurophysiology*, 115, 316–319.

Forsgren, L., Bucht, G., Eriksson, S., et al. (1996). Incidence and clinical characterisation of unprovoked seizures in adults: a prospective population-based study. *Epilepsia*, 37, 224–229.

Forstl, H., Burns, A., Levy, R., et al. (1992). Neurologic signs in Alzheimer's disease: results of a prospective clinical and neuropathologic study. *Archives of Neurology*, 49, 1038–1042.

Gaitatzis, A., Carroll, K., Majeed, A., et al. (2004). The epidemiology of the comorbidity of epilepsy in the general population. *Epilepsia*, 45, 1613–1622.

Hannah, J.A. (1936). A case of Alzheimer's disease with neuropathological findings. *Canadian Medical Association Journal*, 35, 361–366.

Hauser, W.A., (1992). Seizure disorders: the changes with age. *Epilepsia*, 33, S6–S14.

Hauser, W.A., Morris, M.L., Heston, L.L., et al. (1986). Seizures and myoclonus in patients with Alzheimer's disease. *Neurology*, 36, 1226–1230.

Hauser, W.A., Rich, S.S., Lee, J.R., et al. (1998). Risk of recurrent seizures after two unprovoked seizures. *New England Journal of Medicine*, 338, 429–434.

Hermann, B., Seidenberg, M., Sager, M., et al. (2008). Growing old with epilepsy: the neglected issue of cognitive and brain health in aging and elder persons with chronic epilepsy. *Epilepsia*, 49, 731–740.

Hesdorffer, D., Hauser, W., Annegers, J., et al. (1996). Dementia and adult-onset unprovoked seizures. *Neurology*, 46, 727–730.

Johannsen, P., Christensen. J., Goldstein. H., et al. (1996). Epilepsy in Down syndrome – prevalence in three age groups. *Seizure*, 5, 121–125.

Larner, A.J. (2010). Epileptic seizures in AD patients. *Neuromolecular Medicine*, 12, 71–77.

Lott, I.T. and Lai, F. (1982). Dementia in Downs Syndrome: observations from a neurology clinic. *Applied Research in Mental Retardation*, 3, 233–239.

Lozsadi, D. and Larner, A. (2006). Prevalence and causes of seizures at the time of diagnosis of probable Alzheimer's disease. *Dementia and Geriatric Cognitive Disorders*, 22, 121–124.

Martin, R.C., Griffith, H.R., Faught, E., et al. (2005). Cognitive functioning in community dwelling older adults with chronic partial epilepsy. *Epilepsia*, 46, 298–303.

McAreavey, M., Ballinger, B., Fenton, G. (1992). Epileptic seizures in elderly patients with dementia. *Epilepsia*, 33, 657–660.

McKhann, G., Drachman, D., Folstein, M., et al. (1984). Clinical diagnosis of Alzheimer's disease: Report of the NINCDS-ADRDA Work Group under the auspices of Department of Health and Human Services Task Force on Alzheimer's Disease. *Neurology*, 34, 939–944.

McVicker, R.W., Shanks, O.E., McClelland, R.J. (1994). Prevalence and associated features of epilepsy in adults with Down's Syndrome. *British Journal of Psychiatry*, 164, 528–532.

Mendez, M.F., Catanzarro, P., Doss, R.C., et al. (1994). Seizures in Alzheimer's disease: clinicopathologic study. *Journal of Geriatric Psychiatry and Neurology*, 7, 230–233.

Mendez, M.F., and Lim, G.T. (2003). Seizures in elderly patients with dementia: epidemiology and management. *Drugs Aging*, 20, 791–803.

Motamedi, G., and Meador, K. (2003). Epilepsy and cognition. *Epilepsy & Behaviour*, 4, S25–S38.

Neufeld, M.Y., Tanlianski-Aronov, A., Soffer, D., et al. (2003). Generalised convulsive status epilepticus in Creutzfeldt-Jakob disease. *Seizure*, 12, 403–405.

Noebels, J. (2011). A perfect storm: Converging paths of epilepsy and Alzheimer's dementia intersect in the hippocampal formation. *Epilepsia*, 52, S39–S46.

Ortinski, P., and Meador, K.J. (2004). Cognitive side effects of anti-epileptic drugs. *Epilepsy & Behaviour*, 5, S60–S65.

Palop, J.J., and Mucke, L. (2009). Epilepsy and cognitive impairments in Alzheimer's disease. *Archives of Neurology*, 66, 435–444.

Pugh, M.J., Knoefel, J.E., Mortensen, E.M., et al. (2009). New-onset epilepsy risk factors in older veterans. *Journal of the American Geriatrics Society*, 57, 237–242.

Rabinowicz, A.L., Starkstein, S.E., Leiguarda, R.C., et al. (2000). Transient epileptic amnesia in dementia: a treatable unrecognised cause of episodic amnesic wandering. *Alzheimer Disease and Associated Disorders*, 14, 231–233.

Rao, S.C., Dove, G.D., Cascino, G.D., et al. (2009). Recurrent seizures in patients with dementia: frequency, seizure types and treatment outcome. *Epilepsy Behaviour*, 14, 118–120.

Romanelli, M., Morris, J., Ashkin, K., et al. (1990). Advanced Alzheimer's disease is a risk factor for late-onset seizures. *Archives of Neurology*, 47, 847–850.

Rudman, D., John, A., Mattson, D.E., et al. (1988). Seizure disorder in the men of a Veterans Administration nursing home. *Journal of Clinical Epidemiology*, 41, 393–399.

Scarmeas, N., Honig, L., Choi, H., et al. (2009). Seizures in Alzheimer's disease. Who, when and how common? *Archives of Neurology*, 66, 992–997.

Velez-Pardo, C., Arellano, J.I., Cardona-Gomez, P., et al. (2004). CA1 hippocampal loss in familial Alzheimer's Disease Presenilin-1 E280A mutation is related to epilepsy. *Epilepsia*, 45, 751–756.

Volicer, L., Smith, S., Volicer, B. (1995). Effect of seizures on progression of dementia of the Alzheimer type. *Dementia*, 6, 258–263.

Weiner, M.F., Hynan, L.S., Parikh, B., et al. (2003). Can Alzheimer's disease and dementias with Lewy bodies be distinguished clinically? *Journal of Geriatric Psychiatry and Neurology*, 16, 245–250.

Wieser, H.G., Schindler, K., Zumsteg, D. (2006). EEG in Creutzfeldt-Jakob disease. *Clinical Neurophysiology*, 117, 935–951.

# 5

# Weight loss and nutritional disorders

## Introduction

Weight loss accompanied by malnutrition is one of the major manifestations of Alzheimer's disease (AD), and is also seen in other types of dementia. Alois Alzheimer mentioned this particular manifestation of the disease in the case report of his second patient, "Johann F." Alzheimer noted "his body-weight falls slowly and steadily" (1911), and this weight loss as a symptom is consistent with the diagnosis of AD according to the criteria defined by the National Institute of Neurological and Communicative Disorders and Stroke/Alzheimer's Disease and Related Disorders Association (NINCDS–ADRDA) Work Group (McKhann et al., 1984).

The importance of weight loss as a significant comorbidity has been increasingly recognized over the past 25 years (Cronin-Stubbs et al., 1997). One of the early studies by Singh and colleagues (1988) described the problem in a comparative case series, which showed that in a group of hospitalized older women in the UK, those with AD weighed on average 21% less than patients without dementia, and 14% less than those patients with vascular dementia (Singh et al., 1988). Since then many researchers have considered the problem and have shown that malnutrition increases morbidity and mortality, as a loss of muscle mass leads to reduced overall function, resulting in an increase in falls, fractures, decubitus ulcers, and infections (Gillette-Guyonnet et al., 2000).

## The impact of dementia on weight and nutrition

Whereas involuntary weight loss is occasionally reported by older patients without dementia in the context of acute or chronic disease, AD and the other dementias are often accompanied and exacerbated by malnutrition (Magri and Borza, 2003, Faxen-Irving et al., 2005). Many studies have identified low body weight, thinness, and weight loss as clinical characteristics of patients with dementia, and in particular those with AD, especially in the later stages of the disease process (Singh et al., 1988, Burns et al., 1989, Renvall et al., 1989, 1993, Berlinger and Potter, 1991, Faxen-Irving et al., 2002, Guerin et al., 2005b). Indeed, weight loss is considered by many to be one of the principal manifestations of AD (Gillette-Guyonnet et al., 2007). Patients with vascular dementia and frontotemporal dementia (FTD) are also reported to experience weight loss and malnutrition (Liu et al., 2004), as are older people with Down syndrome (Prasher et al., 2004).

Even at an early stage in the disease process, weight changes may become apparent (Claggett, 1989, Niskanen et al., 1993, Renvall et al., 1993, Guyonnet et al., 1998, Guerin et al., 2005a, 2005b, Burns et al., 2010), and weight loss may even precede the diagnosis of dementia (Barrett-Connor et al., 1996, 1998, Knopman et al., 2007). Although some explanations have been offered for the occurrence of weight loss and malnourishment, sometimes in the presence of adequate food intake, the mechanisms still remain unclear. Alterations in eating patterns may contribute to weight loss and may vary with the type of dementia. Such changes in eating patterns may include a reduction in food intake or an increased food intake (Ikeda et al., 2002), although the latter is less common (Morris and Hope, 1989).

Malnutrition is a problem in many nursing-home residents. A study of all Helsinki nursing homes by Suominen and colleagues (2005) found malnutrition in 29% of residents. They identified dementia as an important predictor of malnutrition, among other patient-related factors, including impaired activities of daily living (ADL) and swallowing difficulties. Eating half or less from the food offered in the care facility also had predictive value (Suominen et al., 2005). The issue of nursing homes having adequate staffing levels to provide assistance with eating for people with dementia was highlighted by Woo and colleagues (2005). They examined the prevalence of poor nutrition in residential-care facilities in Hong Kong, and found a higher incidence of poor nutrition (as evidenced by a body mass index (BMI) below 18.5 kg/m$^2$) in facilities with lower staffing levels. A study by Berkhout and colleagues (1998) investigating weight loss in residents in a large Dutch nursing home showed residents with dementia had lower body weight than other residents without dementia. They also found a very strong relationship between weight loss and the inability to choose food and take it to the mouth (seen particularly in residents with dementia).

A very interesting finding confirmed by a number of investigators is that weight loss may precede the diagnosis of dementia by up to 20 years. In a prospective study of 299 patients initially without dementia conducted over 22 years, Barrett-Connor and colleagues reported that subjects later diagnosed with AD had a significant loss of weight between the baseline visit and the diagnosis of dementia being made (Barrett-Connor et al., 1996, 1998). In 2005, Buchman and colleagues reported their findings from a large prospective study of 918 older men, showing that as BMI decreases, the risk of AD increases (Buchman et al., 2005). Similarly the Honolulu–Asia Aging Study showed that in a 32-year prospective study, weight loss began in the years prior to the diagnosis of dementia (Stewart et al., 2005), was independent of confounding factors, and was not seen in those men who had not developed dementia at that stage of follow-up. The majority of the men had lost at least 5 kg in weight prior to the diagnosis of dementia being made. In a study of 449 subjects who were initially without dementia, Johnson and colleagues (2006) reported an overall weight loss among subjects of approximately 0.5 kg per year, which then doubled in subjects who went on to develop dementia, in the 1 or 2 years prior to diagnosis. Finally, in a case–control study, Knopman and colleagues (2007) found that weight loss preceded the diagnosis of dementia in women, but not men, by 20 years or less.

## Epidemiology and prevalence of weight loss in dementia

White and her colleagues (1996) explored the association between AD and weight loss in a study over several years of 362 older people with dementia compared with 317 control subjects. They reported that almost twice as many subjects with AD experienced a weight loss of 5% or more when compared with control subjects, with an overall tendency toward weight loss for both subjects with AD and controls. In a multivariate model, having AD remained a significant predictor for losing 5% or more of body weight in the following year. A follow-up study showed that subjects with AD continued to lose weight at a significantly faster rate than controls, and that the risk of weight loss tended to increase with the severity and progression of the dementia (White et al., 1998). Weight loss was found to be a predictor of mortality, whereas weight gain appeared to have a protective effect.

In a study examining weight loss and energy intake in patients with AD, Wang and colleagues (2004) showed that people with AD were significantly thinner than control subjects, with a poorer appetite and less physical activity, despite having a similar or greater caloric intake than controls. In a multivariate analysis, the presence of AD combined with a poor appetite was the significant predictor of weight loss.

A prospective study of 76 patients with mild to moderate AD showed that almost half the patients experienced more than 4% weight loss in one year, and 13% lost more than 10% of their body weight in a year (Guyonnet et al., 1998). In a larger prospective study of 395 patients with AD, Guerin and colleagues (2005a) reported similar findings, with a third of patients losing at least 4% of their body weight in a year, and 13% of patients losing more than 10% of their body weight in a year.

## Causes of weight loss and malnutrition in dementia

Although it is well established that weight loss accompanies dementia, there is still a lack of understanding about the mechanism for it. It is important to understand the reasons behind this weight loss, as some of these factors may be amenable to treatment, and those factors that are reversible should be identified and addressed. A number of hypotheses to explain weight loss have been put forward, including decreased patient dietary intake due to changes in eating patterns or the ability to feed themselves, an increased energy expenditure, behavioral disturbances, biological changes, or structural changes in the brain (Gillette-Guyonnet et al., 2007). The presence of the APOE-epsilon4 allele has been noted by one group as contributing to weight loss in older women with Alzheimer's disease, with weight loss of more than 5% being found to occur more frequently in those carrying the epsilon4 allele (Vanhanen et al., 2001). A cross-sectional study by Burns and colleagues (2010) suggested that the loss of lean muscle mass is accelerated in older people with AD compared with those without AD. It is unclear whether this loss of muscle is a direct result of dementia pathophysiology, or whether there are underlying shared mechanisms between dementia and sarcopenia (age-related loss of muscle).

## Disordered eating patterns and alteration in dietary intake

Some of the weight and nutritional changes of dementia may be attributable to changes in eating patterns. This may occur early in the development of the disease, particularly in people who live alone. Difficulties with shopping and cooking due to declining abilities in ADL may result in a decreased dietary intake (Riviere et al., 1998), and the loss of previously learned skills has similarly been shown to negatively impact dietary intake (Holm and Soderhamn, 2003). In people with AD who have a caregiver, the higher the level of burden experienced by that caregiver the more likely it is that the person with dementia will experience weight loss (Gillette-Guyonnet et al., 2000, Riviere et al., 2002). It is suggested that these caregivers are simply unable to provide an adequate diet for both the person with dementia and for themselves, due to tiredness or a lack of knowledge (Guyonnet et al., 1998).

In a case–control study by Knopman et al. (2007), the authors suggested that factors such as apathy and a loss of initiative, or a loss of olfactory function, might be reasons for the occurrence of weight loss due to inadequate dietary intake. They also identified the loss of limbic and hypothalamic function that occurs in AD as a possible factor contributing to both the changed sense of satiety, and the subtle changes in swallowing often seen in these patients.

Ikeda and colleagues (2002) investigated changes in eating behaviors in 91 patients with FTD and AD, using a caregiver questionnaire examining the five domains of swallowing problems, food preferences, eating habits, appetite change, and other oral behaviors. They found that changes in eating behaviors were significantly more common in FTD than in AD, with swallowing problems the only symptom that was more common in the AD patients. The authors believed this reflected the involvement of the ventral (orbitobasal) frontal lobe, temporal pole, and amygdala. Eating disorders were also reported as more common in FTD than in AD in a 2004 study by Liu and colleagues (2004). This study reviewed 51 patients with FTD and compared them with 20 normal control subjects and 22 patients with AD. They found that patients with the frontal variant of FTD experienced eating disorders more commonly than those with the temporal variant or those with AD, and related the general increase in behavioral disorders to structural changes in the frontal and temporal lobes.

## Behavioral symptoms

Behavioral symptoms appear to have some effect on weight loss and nutrition. Depression and apathy are implicated as causes of decreased food intake in patients with dementia, and other symptoms such as an increased tendency for distraction, anxiety, and agitation are also significant (Gillette-Guyonnet et al., 2007). Guerin and colleagues studied 393 people with dementia from the REAL.FR cohort (Réseau sur la Maladie d'Alzheimer Français) over a 1-year period (Guerin et al., 2005b). They divided their subjects into three groups based on nutritional status at baseline, and studied cognitive and behavioral characteristics. Those people with the highest occurrence of behavioral symptoms at 1 year of follow-up were in the group with the lowest nutritional status.

In another smaller study, White and colleagues (2004) also showed an association between weight loss and the presence of behavioral symptoms such as agitation, anxiety, and disinhibited behavior, gathered over a 6-month study of 24 patients with dementia in a nursing-home setting. Greenwood and colleagues examined the association between the food intake of 32 people with AD residing in a nursing home, and their cognitive and behavioral symptoms (Greenwood et al., 2005). She showed that the presence of psychomotor disturbances (which included agitation, anxiety, and disinhibition) in residents predicted a decreased protein intake. The study did not examine weight loss over the 2-month period of the study.

In an observational study of residents with dementia in two nursing homes, Pasman and associates (2003) drew attention to the experiences of residential-care nurses managing "food refusal" issues with patients, as can occur in moderately severe dementia. These issues included keeping the mouth shut, or turning the head away when food is offered.

A number of changes in feeding behavior occurs later in the disease process and can be divided into four areas (Gillette-Guyonnet et al., 2007). These include: food selection behaviors, in which there is preference for one type of food over another and a refusal to eat certain foods; an active resistance to feeding and the spitting out of food; feeding dyspraxia, in which there is an inability to use implements or to know how to put food into the mouth; and dysphagia, in which there is a change in, or loss of, the ability to chew and swallow food.

Not all studies have confirmed these findings, and a prospective study of 395 patients with AD examining progressive weight loss and severe weight loss (Guerin et al., 2005a) did not confirm the presence of behavioral symptoms to be a significant cause of progressive weight loss. A study by Lin and colleagues (2010) of almost 500 nursing-home residents with dementia found that a third of these residents had a low food intake at mealtimes. They found a number of major contributory factors – namely a lack of assistance at mealtimes, eating difficulties, and fewer family visits – to decreased food intake in residential aged care facilities. The presence of behavioral problems was not identified as a major problem.

## Increased energy requirements in dementia

One explanation for the weight loss seen in people with dementia is that there exists a hyperbolic state in which energy requirements increase because of the dementia itself (Wang, 2002). In a case–control study of patients with AD, Wang and colleagues found that there was increased weight loss in AD patients compared with controls, despite these patients actually having a higher calorie intake (per kg of body weight per day) than the control patients. They suggested that there was a pathophysiological process in AD that resulted in changes to the metabolic state of these patients. This concept was also investigated a decade earlier by Niskanen and colleagues (1993), who measured resting energy expenditure in older female patients with AD and vascular dementia, using older women without dementia as controls. They demonstrated that there was no difference in energy expenditure at rest between the three groups when adjusted for body weight and lean body mass. Similarly, Donaldson and colleagues (1996) showed no difference in resting metabolic rate between patients with AD and control subjects. Poehlman and colleagues (1997) also found no significant difference in energy expenditure between patients with AD and controls, and in a further study showed that in patients with AD where there was increased physical activity, increased energy intake was associated with increased appendicular skeletal muscle mass (Poehlman and Dvorak, 2000).

## Structural changes in the brain

The medial temporal lobe is involved in the regulation of eating behavior and weight regulation, and is one of the early parts of the brain to show atrophic changes in AD (Grundman et al., 1996). Using magnetic resonance imaging (MRI) morphometric analysis in a study of 58 patients with AD and 16 healthy controls, Grundman and colleagues showed a significant association between a low BMI in patients with AD and atrophy of the medial temporal cortex. Although atrophy was also seen in other brain regions, only the medial temporal cortex atrophy predicted low body weight. Burns et al. (2010) combined MRI imaging and dual-energy X-ray absorptiometry (DEXA) of 70 controls and 70 dementia subjects, with results suggesting that brain atrophy and loss of muscle occur simultaneously.

The findings of a positron emission tomography (PET) study of patients with AD in 2002 suggested that changes in the anterior cingulate cortex (ACC) may be implicated in lower body weight in this group (Hu et al., 2002). The glucose metabolic ratio in the ACC was found to be significantly lower in patients with a low BMI, with no significant differences found in other brain regions. After adjusting for age, gender, and disease duration, an independent association was found between regional glucose metabolism in the ACC and BMI.

## Dysphagia

Dysphagia (difficulty with swallowing) may be a factor in some cases of malnutrition in dementia, particularly in the later stages of the disease, although swallowing problems have also been identified as occurring relatively early in people with AD (Ikeda et al., 2002). Patients with FTD have also been noted to have dysphagia, affecting their food intake (Langmore et al., 2007). Dysphagia is a common symptom in patients with Parkinson's disease and dementia (Bine et al., 1995), and has been reported as an extrapyramidal side effect of risperidone therapy in a patient with AD (Stewart, 2003). Persistent dysphagia occurring late in dementia may be a predictor of imminent death (Chouinard et al., 1998).

## Concomitant medications including cholinesterase inhibitors

Concomitant medications used by people with dementia may lead to changes in food intake due to various side effects, which can include decreased appetite and anorexia, nausea and vomiting, and dry mouth. Cholinesterase inhibitors are indicated for the treatment of mild to moderate AD, but possible gastrointestinal side effects of these medications include anorexia, vomiting, or diarrhea (Cummings, 2003). Such side effects could contribute to weight loss and the development of malnutrition through a reduction in dietary intake. This observation was made by Stewart and Gorelik (2006), who reported weight loss in eight patients on cholinesterase inhibitors. The patients regained weight after the cessation of these medications.

By contrast, cholinesterase inhibitors have demonstrated possible weight-protective properties in other studies, with Guerin and colleagues showing a decreased weight loss in patients taking cholinesterase inhibitors compared with those not taking these medications (Guerin et al., 2005a). Gillette-Guyonnet et al. (2005) also demonstrated that the risk of weight loss was significantly decreased in patients on cholinesterase inhibitors after 1 year of treatment compared with non-treated patients. Similar findings were reported by Vellas and colleagues (2005), who showed that in a study of 530 patients with AD, those patients at risk of poor nutrition showed a greater tendency to gain weight on cholinesterase inhibitors than did well-nourished patients.

## Intervention and management for weight loss and malnutrition

It is important to consider active intervention to prevent and treat malnutrition in patients with dementia in order to prevent the consequences of poor nutrition. These consequences include reduced muscle strength, an increased risk of falls, loss of independence, an increased risk of decubitus ulceration, impaired immunity and an increased chance of infection, and greater risk of death (Gillette-Guyonnet et al., 2000). Weight gain in patients with dementia has been shown to decrease morbidity and increase survival (Keller et al., 2006).

## Assessment

The accurate detection of malnourished patients or those at risk of malnutrition is important. Bedard and colleagues suggested that clinicians may not properly identify potentially malnourished patients on the basis of BMI alone (Bedard et al., 2000), and weight change as measured by regular weight measurement is instead recommended as the optimal way to detect patients at risk of malnutrition (Belmin and EPOC, 2007). It is also recommended that a Mini Nutritional Assessment (MNA) be conducted for patients considered at risk. Those patients at greater risk of weight loss require closer monitoring of their food intake and weight (Inelmen, 2009). Secondary conditions that may affect the ability to eat need to be addressed, such as (and in particular) the dentition of the patient. Using pain relief medication before eating may improve hand and upper limb function where arthritis is a problem (Amella, 2004), and the use of regular oral fluids or artificial saliva may assist in the management of a dry mouth and improve food intake (Holm and Soderhamn, 2003).

In choosing an appropriate mode of intervention to address a patient's weight loss, it is clearly important to assess where the difficulties with nutrition are occurring. The use of a simple assessment tool such as the Eating Behavior Scale may assist in this assessment (Tully et al., 1997). This scale considers six areas of functional ability in eating, which include "able to initiate eating," "able to maintain attention to meal", "able to locate all food," "able to use utensils appropriately," "able to bite, chew, and swallow food without choking," and "able to terminate meal." Correctly identifying the area of difficulty allows for the specific tailoring of management.

## Nutritional supplementation

There is evidence from a number of studies that targeted nutritional interventions are effective in addressing poor nutrition and weight loss (Boffelli et al., 2004). A small study conducted by Faxen-Irving and colleagues (2002) of patients with dementia in residential care found that combining oral supplementation with staff education resulted in weight gain for patients. Gil Gregorio and associates (2003) also demonstrated that nutritional supplements given to nursing-home patients with moderately severe dementia improved their nutritional status and reduced morbidity and mortality over a 1-year period. In 2004 Lauque and colleagues conducted a randomized, controlled study for 3 months into the effects of oral nutritional supplements in 91 people with AD. Energy and protein intakes significantly improved in the intervention group, resulting in a significant increase in weight and fat-free mass, the nutritional benefit of which was maintained in the intervention group after the end of the study (Lauque et al., 2004). However, one study by Young and colleagues (2004) of oral supplementation given to 34 older people with AD living in residential care showed that some residents compensated for the increased energy intake from the oral supplement by decreasing their over-all nutritional intake. This was especially evident in those patients with low body weight who would be the most likely candidates for nutritional intervention. This finding was confirmed by Parrott et al. (2006) in a further analysis of the data from Young's study, in which he showed that older people with a low BMI consumed the oral supplement but reduced their other dietary intake, and subsequently did not increase their oral intake again after the cessation of the supplement, thus poten-tially worsening their nutritional status.

## Education

Interventions should include not only the person with dementia but also their carer, as educational interventions with carers of people with dementia have been shown to be effective in reducing psychological morbidity in the carer, and mortal-ity in the person with dementia (Brodaty et al., 1997). Riviere and colleagues (1998) enrolled carers and community-dwelling patients with AD in a nutritional edu-cation program to prevent weight loss. This involved attending nine 1-hour edu-cational sessions on nutrition and associated subjects such as the management of difficult feeding behaviors. As a result of the program, the nutritional status of the intervention group subjects was maintained over 1 year compared with the control group, in which there was a nutritional status decrease, confirming the potential of nutritional information as a tool to prevent weight loss (Riviere et al., 2001).

The education of health-care staff is also important. Suominen and colleagues (2007) developed an educational program on nutrition including education on the MNA for staff in dementia wards in nursing homes. They demonstrated that over a 1-year period residents' mean energy intake had increased by 21% following the delivery of this education program. Faxen-Irving et al. (2002) included the edu-cation of professional carers of people with dementia in his successful program of oral supplementation for people with dementia in residential care.

## Environmental factors

The environment in which eating occurs has also been shown to have an effect on nutritional status. It is important to preserve a homelike environment and to try and retain food-associated rituals such as having a drink before the evening meal, or saying grace or a blessing before eating (Amella, 2004). Reed and associates (2005) conducted an investigation of characteristics associated with low food and fluid intake in residential-care patients with dementia. Improved food and fluid intake was associated with a higher level of staff monitoring, having meals in a public dining room and the presence of "non-institutional" features (e.g., table-cloths) in the environment.

In a systematic review of interventions to improve nutritional intake in people with dementia, Watson and Green (2006) found that environmental factors were important in improving eating. Seating arrangements and table layout appeared to be important, and there was some evidence for the use of background music. Improving the eating environment by including an aquarium in the dining area was trialled in dementia-specific residential-care units with 62 older people with dementia (Edwards and Beck, 2002). A picture of the ocean was used on the dining room wall in the control unit. Significant weight gain occurred in the intervention group, with no gain in the control group over the 16-week period of the trial. The researchers considered that part of the improvement might have been due to people sitting longer at the dining table watching the fish rather than getting up and wandering.

## Targeted approaches

It is important to ensure that the person with dementia has adequate sensory input in order to participate in the meal. Wearing spectacles and a hearing aid will allow for greater levels of social interaction, and ensure the person with dementia will be able to see visual cues and hear what is being said. Being able to see and recognize familiar food may also increase intake (Amella, 2004).

The type of food served has been shown to influence the level of intake. Making changes to the types of meals served to take into account the preferences of patients with dementia is important. This may involve the use of more soft foods or liquids. The use of finger foods is also recommended as a means of helping patients with dementia maintain their weight, as it avoids the need for utensils, with which they may have difficulty (Soltesz and Dayton, 1993). Biernacki and Barratt (2001) described the changes made in the types of food offered in a long-term care facility for people with dementia. Using finger food, avoiding supplements in cardboard boxes or cans, and the use of familiar food with less of an emphasis on "healthy" foods led to an increased food intake. Decorating food to make it look more interesting and attractive has also been suggested as a method to improve dietary intake (Cohen, 1994).

The timing of meals and supplements is also important. Young and colleagues (2001) studied food intake and behavioral symptoms in 25 older people with AD. They found that the highest energy intake occurred in the morning, consequently recommending that for patients with dementia who had low BMIs, their main food intake should be in the morning period, rather than at more traditional mealtimes. The suggestion has been made that making finger food available throughout the day may also assist in increasing total food intake rather than relying on most eating occurring at mealtimes (Biernacki and Barratt, 2001). Cohen (1994) also suggested maximizing food intake in the early part of the day when cognition is better, and allowing plenty of time for eating.

The use of a comprehensive multifactorial intervention strategy to prevent weight loss in people with dementia has been shown to be effective in a controlled trial in two residential-care facilities. Keller and colleagues (2003) showed that the involvement of a dietitian and development of an individualized eating plan for people with dementia resulted in significant weight gains. Keller extended this work further with the implementation of meal rounds in residential-care facilities (Keller et al., 2006). This involves the direct observation of patients with dementia at mealtimes, with any issues detected subsequently addressed through intervention. Interventions may include changing the form or content of food to address patient preferences, changing the seating arrangement, changing the utensils used, and managing behavioral problems.

Where dysphagia is occurring, interventions need to be tailored toward the cause, although these may be less effective in the more severe stages of dementia. Logemann and colleagues (2008) trialed several interventions for dysphagia in patients with dementia, and in patients with Parkinson's disease. They found the most effective means of preventing the aspiration of thin liquids was through the use of honey-thickened liquids, although patients generally preferred the postural change intervention (chin-down posture). In more severe cases of dementia, none of the interventions was effective.

Physical activity fulfills an important role in maintaining nutritional intake and lean body mass in people with dementia in its capacity to stimulate appetite and prevent muscle from wasting. Dvorak and Poehlman (1998) conducted a case–control study of community-dwelling patients with AD, examining muscle mass, physical activity level, and energy intake. They found that higher levels of physical activity were associated with increased energy intake as well as higher skeletal muscle mass in AD patients. They suggested that physical activity may stimulate energy intake, and the performance of physical activity may assist in the maintenance of good nutritional intake and muscle mass. However, Rolland and colleagues (2007) did not find any change in nutritional status, as measured using the MNA in a 12-month controlled trial of exercise in people with dementia in residential-care facilities.

Special attention needs to be paid to the nutrition of people with dementia admitted to an acute hospital, as demonstrated in an observational study by Miller and colleagues (2006). They showed that patients with a lower limb fracture and cognitive impairment in the orthopedic ward of an acute hospital were at high risk of not achieving adequate protein or energy intake compared with patients without cognitive impairment. They recommended the use of oral nutritional supplementation as a routine treatment for these patients.

## Enteral feeding

The use of enteral nutrition in late-stage dementia remains controversial. Nasogastric feeding tubes and percutaneous endoscopic gastrostomy (PEG) tubes have been used with the aim of improving nutrition and preventing aspiration in patients with severe dysphagia (Sanders et al., 2004). A number of studies have shown decreased survival in patients with dementia and feeding tubes. Additionally, the use of feeding tubes has not been shown to reduce the risk of aspiration pneumonia, malnutrition, or decubitus ulceration (Finucane et al., 1999, Dharmarajan et al., 2001).

A review of 150 community-dwelling patients with neurodegenerative diseases (including dementia) who had received a PEG tube reported limited evidence that

PEG tubes improved functional, nutritional, or subjective health status in this group of patients (Callahan et al., 2000). Similarly, in a retrospective review of 361 patients who had a PEG tube inserted, Sanders and colleagues (2000) found that patients with dementia and a PEG tube had a significantly worse prognosis than those who had a PEG tube inserted for other conditions, with 54% of dementia patients having died at 1 month follow-up, and 90% having died by the end of 1 year. In an observational study of 67 older people with dementia, Alvarez-Fernandez and colleagues (2005) showed that in those patients with advanced dementia the use of a nasogastric tube to provide nutrition actually reduced survival.

Careful hand-feeding of patients with severe dementia with appropriate food may be more effective than enteral feeding. A randomized trial of hand-feeding versus tube-feeding has been suggested to help evaluate the effectiveness of tube-feeding and to provide evidence to inform decisions surrounding its use (DeLegge, 2009). The most recent Cochrane systematic review on the subject of enteral feeding in patients with advanced dementia concluded that there is insufficient evidence to show that enteral feeding is beneficial in patients with dementia (Sampson et al., 2009). Patient and family preferences should be sought before making a feeding decision, and the support of a palliative care specialist is recommended (Buiting et al., 2011).

## Recommendations for the diagnosis and management of weight loss in dementia

Belmin and colleagues (2007) have developed a comprehensive set of consensus guidelines for the diagnosis and management of weight loss in AD based on a literature review and consensus development approach. The following recommendations are extracted from those guidelines:

1. In patients with dementia, nutritional status should be assessed at the time of diagnosis and/or the start of treatment. This should include measurement of body weight and an MNA carried out with the help of a family caregiver.
2. Body weight should be measured and recorded monthly, and on visits to the treating physician.
3. Initiation of a nutritional intervention should occur if two or more of the following are present:
   a. MNA score <17
   b. plasma albumin <35 g/L
   c. decrease in food intake assessed over 3 days
   d. loss of more than 5% of body weight over 6 months.
4. A nutritional intervention should include:
   a. a search for reversible medical or socio-environmental causes for intake reduction
   b. increased calorie/protein intake (oral supplementation by food and/or by dietary supplements)
   c. daily physical activity.

5. If situations involving medical stress occur, such as surgery or severe infection, nutritional support should be provided.
6. To improve food intake consider the use of finger foods, favorite foods, home-like environment (e.g., tablecloths), and background music, and give oral supplements 2 hours before meals rather than with meals.
7. Education of family and professional caregivers in management of weight loss and use of nutritional interventions may be beneficial.
8. Enteral feeding in late-stage dementia is unlikely to be effective.

---

### Case studies

Mr. K is an 82-year-old man with moderate AD. He lives with his wife in their own home. He had been gradually losing weight, beginning approximately 3 years before his diagnosis was made. His wife said that her husband enjoyed his food, but no matter how much she fed him Mr. K continued to slowly lose weight. He was reviewed by a dietitian, who gave him a pedometer to measure daily walking activity, and Mrs. D completed a food diary for 1 month. The pedometer showed that Mr. K was not overly physically active, and he was consuming a well-balanced diet of approximately 2500 kcals each day. The dietitian suggested that Mr. K add a tin of high-protein high-calorie nutritional supplement after breakfast and lunch each day. Mr. K was able to tolerate the supplement without significantly reducing his daily food intake. His weight stabilized over the following 3 months and dropped only minimally over the next 6 months.

Mrs. Y is a retired, 54-year-old lawyer who lives with her husband. She has moderately severe FTD, and has had a classical pattern of stereotyped eating behavior with a predilection for sweet foods. Previously a fitness fanatic, her weight was now increasing signficantly. She would eat the same food for every meal, ice cream and fruit salad, and became fixated on chocolate, constantly scanning her environment for more possible supplies. As she responded impulsively to her environment, her husband cleared all foods from her view, and tried to have her exercise with him. These strategies have had limited success.

---

### Key points

- People with Alzheimer's disease may lose up to 10% of body weight during the course of the disease. People with vascular dementia and frontotemporal dementia are also likely to lose weight.
- Weight loss may occur up to 20 years before the appearance of cognitive symptoms.

> • Dementia patients at risk of weight loss and malnutrition should be iden-
> tified and treated to prevent loss of muscle mass and strength, pres-
> sure ulcers, and loss of immunity with subsequently increased rate of
> infection.

## References

Alvarez-Fernandez, B.M.A., Garcia-Ordonez, Martinez-Manzaneres, C., Gomez-
Heulgas, R. (2005). Survival of a cohort of elderly patients with advanced
dementia: nasogastric tube feeding as a risk factor for mortality. *International
Journal of Geriatric Psychiatry*, 20, 363–370.

Alzheimer, A. (1911). Uber eingenartige Krankeitsfalle des spateren Alters [on
certain peculiar diseases of old age]. *Zeitsschrift fur die gesamte Neurologie und
Psychiatrie*, 4, 356–385.

Amella, E.J. (2004). Feeding and hydration issues for older adults with dementia.
[Erratum appear in Nurs Clin North Am (2006). 41, 129]. *Nursing Clinics of
North America*, 39, 607–623.

Barrett-Connor, E., Edelstein, S., Corey-Bloom, J., Wiederholt, W. (1996). Weight
loss precedes dementia in community-dwelling older adults. *Journal of the
American Geriatrics Society*, 44, 1147–1152.

Barrett-Connor, E., Edelstein, S., Corey-Bloom, J., Wiederholt, W. (1998).
Weight loss precedes dementia in community-dwelling older adults. *Journal of
Nutrition, Health & Aging*, 2, 113–114.

Bedard, M., Molloy, D.W., Bell, R., Lever, J. (2000). Determinants and detection of
low body mass index in community-dwelling adults with Alzheimer's disease.
*International Psychogeriatrics*. 12, 87–98.

Belmin, J. and Expert Panel and Organisation Committee. (2007). Practical guidelines for the diagnosis and management of weight loss in Alzheimer's disease:
a consensus from appropriateness ratings of a large expert panel. *Journal of
Nutrition, Health & Aging*, 11, 33–37.

Berkhout, A.M., Cools, H.J., van Houwelingen H.C. (1998). The relationship
between difficulties in feeding oneself and loss of weight in nursing-home
patients with dementia. *Age & Ageing*, 27, 637–641.

Berlinger, W.G. and Potter, J.F. (1991). Low Body Mass Index in demented outpatients. *Journal of the American Geriatrics Society*, 39, 973–978.

Biernacki, C. and J. Barratt. (2001). Improving the nutritional status of people
with dementia. *British Journal of Nursing*, 10, 1104–1114.

Bine, J.E., Frank, E.M., McDade, H.L. (1995). Dysphagia and dementia in subjects
with Parkinson's disease. *Dysphagia*, 10, 160–164.

Boffelli, S., Rozzini, R., Trabucchi, M. (2004). Nutritional intervention in special care
units for dementia. *Journal of the American Geriatrics Society*, 52, 1216–1217.

Brodaty, H., Gresham, M., Luscombe, G. (1997). The Prince Henry Hospital
dementia caregiver's training programme. *International Journal of Geriatric
Psychiatry*, 12, 183–192.

Buchman, A.S., Wilson, R.S., Bienas, J.L., Shah, R.C., Evans, D.A., Bennett, D.A. (2005). Change in body mass index and risk of incident Alzheimer disease. *Neurology*, 65, 892–897.

Buiting, H., Clayton, J., Butow, P., et al. (2011). Artificial nutrition and hydration for patients with advanced dementia: perspectives from medical practitioners in the Netherlands and Australia. *Palliative Medicine*, 25, 83–91.

Burns, A., Marsh, A., Bender, D. (1989). Dietary intake and clinical, anthropometric and biochemical indices of malnutrition in elderly demented patients and non-demented subjects. *Psychological Medicine*, 19, 383–391.

Burns, J., Johnson, D., Watts, A., Swerdlow, R., Brooks, W. (2010). Reduced lean mass in early alzheimer disease and its association with brain atrophy. *Archives of Neurology*, 67, 428–433.

Callahan, C., Haeg, K., Weinburger, M. (2000). Outcomes of PEG amongst older adults in a community setting. *Journal of the American Geriatrics Society* 48, 1048–1054.

Chouinard, J., Lavigne, E., Villeneuve, C. (1998). Weight loss, dysphagia, and outcome in advanced dementia. *Dysphagia*, 13, 151–155.

Claggett, M.S. (1989). Nutritional factors relevant to Alzheimer's disease. *Journal of the American Dietetic Association*, 89, 392–396.

Cohen, D. (1994). Dementia, depression, and nutritional status. *Primary Care* 21, 107–119.

Cronin-Stubbs, D., Beckett, L.A., Scherr, P., et al. (1997). Weight loss in people with Alzheimer's disease: a prospective population based analysis. *British Medical Journal*, 314, 178–9.

Cummings, J.L. (2003). Use of cholinesterase inhibitors in clinical practice: Evidence-based recommendations. *American Journal of Geriatric Psychiatry*, 11, 131–145.

DeLegge, M. (2009). Tube feeding in patients with dementia: where are we? *Nutrition in Clinical Practice*, 24, 214–216.

Dharmarajan, T.S., Unnikrishnan, D., Pitchumoni, C.S. (2001). Percutaneous endoscopic gastrostomy and outcome in dementia. *American Journal of Gastroenterology*, 96, 2556–2563.

Donaldson, K.E., Carpenter, W.H., Toth, M.J., Goran, M.J., Newhouse, P., Poehlman, E.T. (1996). No evidence for a higher resting metabolic rate in non-institutionalized Alzheimer's disease patients. *Journal of the American Geriatrics Society*, 44, 1232–1234.

Dvorak, R.V. and Poehlman, E.T. (1998). Appendicular skeletal muscle mass, physical activity, and cognitive status in patients with Alzheimer's disease. *Neurology*, 51, 1386–1390.

Edwards, N. and Beck, A. (2002). Animal-assisted therapy and nutrition in Alzheimer's disease. *Western Journal of Nursing Research*, 24, 697–712.

Faxen-Irving, G., Andren-Olsson, B., af Geijerstam, A., Basun, H., Cederholm, T. (2002). The effect of nutritional intervention in elderly subjects residing in group-living for the demented. *European Journal of Clinical Nutrition*, 56, 221–227.

Faxen-Irving, G., Basun, H., Cederholm, T. (2005). Nutritional and cognitive relationships and long-term mortality in patients with various dementia disorders. *Age & Ageing*, 34, 136–141.

Finucane, T.E., Christmas, C., Travis K. (1999). Tube feeding in patients with advanced dementia: a review of the evidence. *Journal of the American Medical Association*, 282, 1365–1370.

Gil Gregorio, P., Ramirez Diaz, S.P., Ribera Casado, J.M., Demenu Group. (2003). Dementia and Nutrition. Intervention study in institutionalized patients with Alzheimer disease. Journal of Nutrition, *Health & Aging*, 7, 304–308.

Gillette-Guyonnet, S., Abellan Van Kan, G., Andrieu, S., et al. (2007). IANA (International Academy on Nutrition and Aging) Expert Group: weight loss and Alzheimer's disease. *Journal of Nutrition, Health & Aging*, 11, 38–48.

Gillette-Guyonnet, S., Cortes, F., Cantet, C., Vellas, B., The REAL.FR Group. (2005). Long-term cholinergic treatment is not associated with greater risk of weight loss during Alzheimer's disease: data from the French REAL.FR cohort. *Journal of Nutrition, Health & Aging*, 9, 69–73.

Gillette-Guyonnet, S., Nourhashemi, F., Andrieu, S., et al. (2000). Weight loss in Alzheimer disease. *American Journal of Clinical Nutrition*, 71, 637S–642S.

Greenwood, C., Tam, C., Chen, M., Young, K., Binns, M., van Reekum, R. (2005). Behavioural disturbances not cognitive deterioration are associated with altered food selection in seniors with Alzheimer's disease. *Journal of Gerontology*, 60A, 499–505.

Grundman, M., Corey-Bloom, J., Jernigan, T., Archibald, S., Thal, L. (1996). Low body weight in Alzheimer's disease is associated with mesial temporal cortex atrophy. *Neurology*, 46, 1585–1591.

Guerin, O., Andrieu, S., Schneider, S., et al. (2005a). Different modes of weight loss in Alzheimer disease: a prospective study of 395 patients. *American Journal of Clinical Nutrition*, 82, 435–441.

Guerin, O., Soto, M. E., Brocker, P., et al. (2005b). Nutritional status assessment during Alzheimer's disease: results after one year (the REAL French Study Group). *Journal of Nutrition, Health & Aging*, 9, 81–84.

Guyonnet, S., Nourhashemi, F., Ousset, P.J., et al. (1998). Factors associated with weight loss in Alzheimer's disease. *Journal of Nutrition, Health & Aging*, 2, 107–109.

Holm, B., and Soderhamn, O. (2003). Factors associated with nutritional status in a group of people in an early stage of dementia. *Clinical Nutrition*, 22, 385–389.

Hu, X., Okamura, N., Arai, H., et al. (2002) Neuroanatomical correlates of low body weight in Alzheimer's disease: a PET study. *Progress in Neuro-Psychopharmacology & Biological Psychiatry*, 26, 1285–1289.

Ikeda, M., Brown, J., Holland, A., Fukuhara, R., Hodges, J. (2002). Changes in appetite, food preference, and eating habits in frontotemporal dementia and Alzheimer's disease. *Journal of Neurology, Neurosurgery, & Psychiatry*, 73, 371–376.

Inelmen, E., Sergi, G., Coin, A., et al. (2009). An open-ended question: Alzheimer's disease and involuntary weight loss: which comes first? *Aging Clinical and Experimental Research*, 22, 192–197.

Johnson, D.K., Wilkins, C.H., Morris, J.C. (2006). Accelerated weight loss may precede diagnosis in Alzheimer disease. *Archives of Neurology*, 63, 1312–1317.

Keller, H.H., Gibbs A., Boudreau, L., Goy, R.E., Patillo, M.S., Brown, H.M. (2003). Prevention of weight loss in dementia with comprehensive nutritional treatment. *Journal of the American Geriatrics Society*, 51, 945–952.

Keller, H.H., Gibbs-Ward A., Randall-Simpson, J., Bocock, M.A., Dimou, E. (2006). Meal rounds: an essential aspect of quality nutrition services in long-term care. *Journal of the American Medical Directors Association*, 7, 40–45.

Knopman, D.S., Edland, S.D., Cha, R.H., Petersen, R.C., Rocca, W.A. (2007). Incident dementia in women is preceded by weight loss by at least a decade. *Neurology*, 69, 739–746.

Langmore, S.E., Olney, R.K., Lomen-Hoerth, C., Miller, B.L. (2007). Dysphagia in patients with frontotemporal lobar dementia. *Archives of Neurology*, 64, 58–62.

Lauque, S., Arnaud-Battandier, F., Gillette, S., et al. (2004). Improvement of weight and fat-free mass with oral nutritional supplementation in patients with Alzheimer's disease at risk of malnutrition: a prospective randomized study. *Journal of the American Geriatrics Society*, 52: 1702–1707.

Lin, L., Watson, R., Wu, S. (2010). What is associated with low food intake in older people with dementia? *Journal of Clinical Nursing*, 19, 53–59.

Liu, W., Miller, B. L., Kramer, J.H., et al. (2004). Behavioral disorders in the frontal and temporal variants of frontotemporal dementia. *Neurology*, 62, 742–748.

Logemann, J.A., Gensler, G., Robbins, J., et al. (2008). A randomized study of three interventions for aspiration of thin liquids in patients with dementia or Parkinson's disease. *Journal of Speech Language & Hearing Research*, 51, 173–183.

Magri, F. and Borza, A. (2003). Nutritional assessment of demented patients: a descriptive study. *Aging-Clinical & Experimental Research*, 15, 148–153.

McKhann, G., Drachman, D., Folstein, M., et al. (1984). Clinical diagnosis of Alzheimer's disease: report of the NINCDS-ADRDA Work Group. *Neurology*, 34, 939–944.

Miller, M.D., Bannerman, E., Daniels, L., Crotty, M. (2006). Lower limb fracture, cognitive impairment and risk of subsequent malnutrition: a prospective evaluation of dietary energy and protein intake on an orthopaedic ward. *European Journal of Clinical Nutrition*, 60, 853–861.

Morris, C.H., and Hope, R.A. (1989). Eating habits in dementia. A descriptive study. *British Journal of Psychiatry*, 154, 801–806.

Niskanen, L., Piirainen, M., Koljonen, M., Uusituppa, M. (1993). Resting energy expenditure in relation to energy intake in patients with Alzheimer's disease, multi-infarct dementia and in control women. *Age & Ageing*, 22, 132–137.

Parrott, M., Young, K., Greenwood, C. (2006). Energy containing nutritional supplements can affect usual energy intake post supplementation. *Journal of the American Geriatrics Society*, 54, 1382–1387.

Pasman, H.R., The, B.A., Onwuteaka-Philipsen, B., van der Wal, G., Ribbe, M. (2003). Feeding nursing home patients with severe dementia: a qualitative study. *Journal of Advanced Nursing*, 42, 304–311.

Poehlman, E.T. and Dvorak, R.V. (2000). Energy expenditure, energy intake, and weight loss in Alzheimer disease. *American Journal of Clinical Nutrition*, 71, 650S–655S.

Poehlman, E.T., Toth, M.J., Goran, M.I. Carpenter, W.H., Newhouse, P., Rosen, C.J. (1997). Daily energy expenditure in free-living non-institutionalized Alzheimer's patients: a doubly labeled water study. *Neurology*, 48, 997–1002.

Prasher, V.P., Metseagharun, T., Hauque, S. (2004). Weight loss in adults with Down syndrome and with dementia in Alzheimer's disease. *Research in Developmental Disabilities*, 25, 1–7.

Reed, P.S., Zimmerman, S., Sloane, P.D., Williams, C.S., Boustani, M. (2005). Characteristics associated with low food and fluid intake in long-term care residents with dementia. *Gerontologist*, 45, 74–80.

Renvall, M.J., Spindler, A.A., Nichols, J.F., Ramsdell, J.W. (1993). Body composition of patients with Alzheimer's disease. *Journal of the American Dietetic Association*, 93, 47–52.

Renvall, M.J., Spindler, A.A., Ramsdell, J.W., Paskvan, M. (1989). Nutritional status of free-living Alzheimer's patients. *American Journal of the Medical Sciences*, 298, 20–27.

Riviere, S., Gillette-Guyonnet, S., Andrieu, S., et al. (2002). Cognitive function and caregiver burden: predictive factors for eating behaviour disorders in Alzheimer's disease. *International Journal of Geriatric Psychiatry*, 17, 950–955.

Riviere, S., Gillette-Guyonnet, S., Voisin, T., et al. (2001). A nutritional education program could prevent weight loss and slow cognitive decline in Alzheimer's disease. *Journal of Nutrition, Health & Aging*, 5, 295–299.

Riviere, S., Lauque, S., Vellas, B. (1998). Health promotion programme: nutrition and Alzheimer's disease. *Journal of Nutrition, Health & Aging*, 2, 101–106.

Rolland, Y., Pillard, F., Klapouszczak, A., et al. (2007). Exercise program for nursing home residents with Alzheimer's disease: a 1-year randomized, controlled trial. *Journal of the American Geriatrics Society*, 55, 158–65.

Sampson, E.L., Candy, B., Jones, L. (2009). Enteral tube feeding for older people with advanced dementia. *Cochrane Database of Systematic Reviews*, 2, CD007209.

Sanders, D.S., Anderson, A.J., Bardhan, K.D. (2004). Percutaneous endoscopic gastrostomy: an effective strategy for gastrostomy feeding in patients with dementia. *Clinical Medicine*, 4, 235–241.

Sanders, D.S., Carter, M.J., D'Silva, J., James, G., Bolton, R.P., Bardhan, K.D. (2000). Survival analysis in percutaneous endoscopic gastrostomy feeding: a worse outcome in patients with dementia. *American Journal of Gastroenterology*, 95, 1472–1475.

Singh, S., Mulley, G.P., Losowsky, M.S. (1988). Why are Alzheimer patients thin? *Age & Ageing*, 17, 21–28.

Soltesz, K., Dayton, J. (1993). Finger foods help those with Alzheimer's disease maintain weight. *Journal of the American Dietetic Association*, 93, 1106–1108.

Stewart, J.T. (2003). Dysphagia associated with risperidone therapy. *Dysphagia*, 18, 274–275.

Stewart, J.T. and Gorelik, A.R. (2006). Involuntary weight loss associated with cholinesterase inhibitors in dementia. *Journal of the American Geriatrics Society*, 54, 1013–1014.

Stewart, R., Masaki, K., Xue, Q.L., et al. (2005). A 32-year prospective study of change in body weight and incident dementia: the Honolulu-Asia Aging Study. *Archives of Neurology*, 62, 55–60.

Suominen, M., Kivisto, S., Pitkala, K. (2007). The effects of nutrition education on professionals' practice and on nutrition of aged residents in dementia wards. *European Journal of Clinical Nutrition*, 61, 1226–1232.

Suominen, M., Muurinen, S., Routasalo, P., et al. (2005). Malnutrition and associated factors among aged residents in all nursing homes in Helsinki. *European Journal of Clinical Nutrition*, 59, 578–583.

Tully, M.W., Lambros Matrakas, K., Muir, J., et al. (1997). The Eating Behaviour Scale: a simple method of assessing functional ability in patients with Alzheimer's disease. *Journal of Gerontological Nursing*, 23, 9–15.

Vanhanen, M., Kivipelto, M., Koivisto, K., et al. (2001). APOE-epsilon4 is associated with weight loss in women with AD: a population-based study. *Neurology*, 56, 655–659.

Vellas, B., Lauque, S., Gillette-Guyonnet, S., et al. (2005). Impact of nutritional status on the evolution of Alzheimer's disease and on response to acetylcholinesterase inhibitor treatment. *Journal of Nutrition, Health & Aging*, 9, 75–80.

Wang, P.N., Yang, C.L., Lin, K.N., Chen, W.T., Chwang, L.C., Liu, H.C. (2004). Weight loss, nutritional status and physical activity in patients with Alzheimer's disease. A controlled study. *Journal of Neurology*, 251, 314–320.

Wang, S.Y. (2002). Weight loss and metabolic changes in dementia. *Journal of Nutrition, Health & Aging*, 6, 201–205.

Watson, R. and Green, S. (2006). Feeding and dementia: a systematic literature review. *Journal of Advanced Nursing*, 54, 86–93.

White, H., Pieper, C., Schmader, K. (1998). The association of weight change in Alzheimer's disease with severity of disease and mortality: a longitudinal analysis. *Journal of the American Geriatrics Society*, 46, 1223–1227.

White, H., Pieper, C., Schmader, K., Fillenbaum, G. (1996). Weight change in Alzheimer's disease. *Journal of the American Geriatrics Society*, 44, 265–272.

White, H.K., McConnell, E.S., Bales, C.W., Kuchibhatla, M. (2004). A 6-month observational study of the relationship between weight loss and behavioral symptoms in institutionalized Alzheimer's disease subjects. *Journal of the American Medical Directors Association*, 5, 89–97.

Woo, J., Chi, I., Hui, E., Chan, F., Sham, A. (2005). Low staffing level is associated with malnutrition in long term residential care homes. *European Journal of Clinical Nutrition*, 59, 474–479.

Young, K.W., Binns, M.A., Greenwood, C.E. (2001). Meal delivery practices do not meet needs of Alzheimer patients with increased cognitive and behavioral difficulties in a long-term care facility. *Journals of Gerontology Series A-Biological Sciences & Medical Sciences*, 56, M656–M661.

Young, K.W., Greenwood, C.E., van Reekum, R., Binns, M.A. (2004). Providing nutrition supplements to institutionalized seniors with probable Alzheimer's disease is least beneficial to those with low body weight status. *Journal of the American Geriatrics Society*, 52, 1305–1312.

# 6

# Incontinence

## Introduction

Incontinence of urine or feces in older age can cause great distress and lead to social isolation. Age-related changes in bladder and bowel function are well documented in the older adult population (Resnick, 1995, Ratnaike et al., 2000, Wilson, 2003, Bravo, 2004, Pringle-Specht, 2005). Physiological aging affects a number of structures within the nervous system, and the lower urinary tract, including the prostate in men and pelvic floor muscles in women, causing changes that make older people more vulnerable to incontinence. These changes alone are not entirely responsible for continence loss; changes to bladder capacity, bladder contractility, and the inability to delay voiding also increase the risk of urinary incontinence.

The increase in the prevalence of urinary incontinence in older adults is largely due to a combination of comorbidities, medication, functional decline, and age-related changes (Jirovic and Templin, 2001, Durrant and Snape, 2003, Wilson, 2003, Bravo, 2004, Ostbye et al., 2004, Fowler, 2006, Sakakibara et al., 2008, Goode et al., 2010, Hägglund, 2010,). Incontinence in the person with dementia is a result of these changes that occur with normal aging, combined with the inability to employ compensatory measures to avoid incontinence owing to cognitive impairment and executive dysfunction (Resnick, 1995, Sakakibara et al., 2008).

## Definitions and physiology of continence

**Urinary incontinence** (UI) may be defined simply as any involuntary leakage of urine (Pinkowski, 1996). UI can be a chronic condition or can present as transient and reversible, as the result of a urinary tract infection, delirium, excessive coughing from a respiratory tract infection, constipation, or medication side effects (Pringle-Specht, 2005). Several types of UI are reported in the literature. These include stress, urge, mixed, obstructive, and overflow incontinence, with the latter two types occurring more frequently in the male population.

**Detrusor hyperactivity** (overactivity of the smooth muscle in the bladder wall) is the most commonly diagnosed cause of UI, and presents as urge incontinence, frequency, and nocturia. Causes can include neurological disorders, bladder disease, medication, and cognitive impairment.

**Stress incontinence** is frequently diagnosed in older women and is related to weak pelvic floor muscles, with leakage occurring simultaneously with intra-abdominal pressure change, for example when coughing or straining.

**Obstruction with overflow** is commonly seen in males with an enlarged prostate gland, but may also result from fecal impaction, medication side effects, and neurological disorders.

**Functional incontinence** is the end result of external influences on continence, and is due to immobility, a lack of environmental support, physical barriers, and cognitive impairment, in the absence of physical dysfunction or disease of the urinary system.

**Fecal incontinence** (FI) is defined as the involuntary passing of liquid or solid stool and can also include incontinence of flatus (Powell and Rigby, 2002). Common causes of FI include constipation and fecal impaction with overflow, acute or chronic diarrhea, previous surgery, and the effects of medication. The reversibility of the incontinence will be determined by the cause of the problem.

**Constipation and fecal impaction with overflow** can result from several factors, including a reduction in dietary fiber, reduced fluid intake, over-the-counter medication, prescription medications, and decreased mobility (Tarqid, 2007, Leung and Rao, 2009).

**Diarrhea** is a common outcome of the overuse of laxatives, some over-the-counter medications containing magnesium or sorbitol, radiation treatment to the lower abdomen, chronic bowel disease, and food-related infections (Tarqid, 2007).

## Physiology of normal bladder control

Voluntary control of urinary function is a complex process and relies on several neural pathways linking the cerebral cortex, pontine micturition centre, spinal cord, sacral nerves, urinary bladder, pelvic floor muscles, and the sphincters (Blok et al., 1997, Fowler, 2006). The cortex and pontine micturition centre control the act of micturition so that it occurs at an appropriate time and place. In particular, the prefrontal cortex plays an important role in planning complex cognitive behavior and appropriate social behavior, both of which are essential in maintaining continence (Wood and Grafman, 2003).

Remaining continent requires a complex interaction of several factors. Jirovec and Wells (1990) have summarized these essential factors to be the presence of an adequate stimulus to initiate the micturition reflex (i.e., a full bladder), the neuro-muscular and structural integrity of the genitourinary system and spinal cord, the cognitive ability to interpret and respond to the sensation of a full bladder, and the motivation to want to inhibit the passage of urine. All of these factors other than a full bladder may be adversely affected by dementia. The individual must also have adequate mobility to enable them to react before the urge to urinate overwhelms the ability to inhibit the urge.

## Epidemiology of incontinence in dementia

Urinary and fecal incontinence are both underreported in the community because of the social stigma and embarrassment experienced by sufferers. FI in particular is a significant cause of embarrassment, with many patients reluctant to report the problem (Kalantar et al., 2002). Prevalence rates of both UI and FI vary greatly within the literature depending on the methodologies and definitions used. Variations are also seen between community-dwelling individuals and nursing-home populations, and in people with and without dementia.

A study of 144 community-dwelling older patients with dementia found that 33% had UI (Miu et al., 2010). A review article by Durrant and Snape (2003) of UI prevalence rates for the United Kingdom and the United States reported that more than 50% of nursing-home residents had UI. The authors noted that nursing-home residents are a heterogeneous group, and with various levels of physical frailty, cognitive impairment, and poor mobility occurring in residents in every facility, direct comparisons between studies were difficult. However, the results from a number of studies do indicate that UI is up to four times more common in people with dementia compared with people without dementia. Yap and Tan (2006) reported a prevalence rate of 13% in people without dementia, compared with a rate of up to 53% in dementia populations. Studies have reported prevalence rates of UI within the older adult population without dementia as between 6 and 14% (Brocklehurst, 1993, Yap and Tan, 2006), whereas Bravo (2004) has reported that UI affects 22% of individuals with dementia living in the community, and up to 84% of nursing-home residents with dementia.

A study by Ouslander et al. (1990) recruited 184 people with dementia and their caregivers living in the community. Alzheimer's disease (AD) accounted for 38% of the study population, whereas 20% were listed as having vascular dementia, and 42% were listed as "other dementia." The mean Mini-Mental State Examination (MMSE) score for continent individuals was 15/30, with the incontinent group recording a mean score of 11/30. The study reported a 36% UI prevalence rate equally divided between males (35%) and females (34%). The authors also noted the frequency of UI increased with age and lower cognitive scores.

In another study, Pringle-Specht and colleagues (2002) surveyed 13 residential-care facilities. The authors recruited a convenience sample of 145 residents with a mean age of 83, and a mean length of stay of 2.65 years in the facility. Two-thirds of the sample was made up of women. In total, 81% of residents were incontinent, with 48% having been incontinent on admission. When incontinence was ana-lyzed in association with primary medical diagnoses, 95% of people in the sample study were shown to have dementia.

# The impact of dementia on continence

Urinary incontinence in dementia occurs at different times in the course of the disease process and with differing frequency, depending on the type of dementia. UI is seen more frequently in AD patients than in patients with vascular dementia, becoming more common as the disease progresses (Davidson et al., 1991, Diehl-Schmid et al., 2007). Upton and Reed (2005) describe incontinence in people with dementia (when not linked to infection) as the result of a progressive dysfunction directly linked to a lack of concentration, insight, judgment, and motivation, in addition to disorientation and general lethargy. Visuospatial difficulties, apraxia, and procedural memory loss can also interfere with the ability to maintain continence, leading to difficulties in performing self-toileting (Knight, 2000, Yap and Tan, 2006). However, in contrast to this functional explanation, Diehl-Schmid and colleagues (2007) put forward a more organic cause of incontinence, suggesting that it is likely to be due to a loss of prefrontal control over voiding reflexes and a loss of sphincter control, both of which are hallmarks of moderate to severe dementia.

As mentioned earlier, there are differences in incontinence rates between the different forms of dementia. A prospective longitudinal study recruited 73 patients with dementia and followed them until death with the performance of a brain autopsy (Del-Ser et al., 1996). All of the participants had well-documented UI, with 29 patients having AD, 11 having diffuse Lewy body disease (DLBD), 13 having Alzheimer's disease with Lewy bodies (AD+LB), and 20 patients having Alzheimer's disease and vascular dementia (AD+VaD). The clinical diagnosis was confirmed by histologic analysis of ten brain regions by a blinded investigator. The study found incontinence occurred as an early marker of VaD, or in AD when associated with vascular lesions. The onset of incontinence was significantly earlier in the DLBD group than in the AD group, with the time to death also shorter in the DLBD group (2.4 years vs. 3.0 years). Patients with AD developed incontinence late in the disease, usually when severe cognitive impairment was present. By contrast, DLBD patients developed incontinence prior to severe cognitive impairment being present.

A small study by Ransmyr et al. (2008) performed urodynamics studies on 15 patients with DLBD, 15 patients with Parkinson's disease (PD), and 16 AD patients referred for assessment of incontinence. The authors confirmed UI is an early symptom of DLBD, whereas in AD it occurs at a more advanced stage of the disease. They also found detrusor overactivity was more frequent in the DLBD patients than in those patients with PD or AD.

Patients with frontotemporal dementia (FTD) were also found to have early-onset UI compared with AD patients. A study by Diehl-Schmid et al. (2007) found that several participants reported incontinence in the early stages of the disease. The authors concluded that given the vast network of cortical and subcortical regions of the brain involved in micturition, patients with FTD may lose both frontal cortical control and social control, resulting in an unstable or overactive bladder, and an inability of the frontal cortex to prevent bladder contractility until a socially acceptable time. A second study in patients with FTD and UI using positron emission tomography (PET) found functional brain alterations in the limbic system in those patients who were incontinent (Perneczky et al., 2008). The limbic system is involved in cognitive function and in executive control, both of which are important elements in maintaining continence.

## Assessment of urinary incontinence

Given that the etiology of incontinence in the person with dementia can be multifactorial, a comprehensive assessment is required to rule out reversible causes of incontinence. A number of causes of incontinence have been identified in the literature as avoidable and reversible. These include delirium, infection, atrophic urethritis and vaginitis, prostatic hypertrophy, medication side effects, excessive urinary output, fecal impaction, restricted mobility, and use of physical restraints (Bravo, 2004, Yap and Tan, 2006, Sakakibara et al., 2008).

It is also recommended that a thorough medical assessment be completed covering the following areas (Resnick, 1995, Wilson, 2003, Bravo, 2004, Hägglund, 2010):

- *medical history*: including the most relevant medical background (diabetes, heart failure, other neurological disorders) and relevant surgical history (urological, gynecological, pelvic surgery)
- *cognitive assessment*: including the severity and type of dementia
- *physical examination*: including rectal examination and pelvic examination
- *medication review*: prescription and over-the-counter medications (diuretics, laxatives, sedative-hypnotics, antipsychotics, antidepressants, analgesics)
- *functional assessment*: of mobility and transfer ability; consider environmental factors limiting access to the toilet
- *history of incontinence*: recency of onset, frequency, history of urinary tract infections, nocturia, urge, stress, retention, overflow, diarrhea
- *laboratory assessments*: including urinalysis, blood count, biochemistry
- *urodynamic studies*: bladder ultrasound to measure post-void residual volume, and consider urodynamic studies if cause of incontinence is unclear.

## Intervention and management for urinary incontinence in dementia

Incontinence in dementia is due to a multifactorial breakdown in compensatory mechanisms, and functional incontinence is believed to be the predominant cause of incontinence in people with dementia (Hutchinson et al., 1996, Gaugler et al., 2009).

It is unlikely that any specific treatment aimed solely at treating incontinence in this group will be available in the near future (Fowler, 2006). The aim instead is to manage incontinence in the best possible way to reduce embarrassment and preserve dignity.

## Prompted voiding programs

Prompted voiding (PV) programs dominate the literature as a management tool for older adults, for those with and without dementia residing in the community or residential care. Given that functional incontinence is common in people with dementia, as the disease precludes the proactive involvement of the person in self-toileting, all PV programs will require the active involvement of a caregiver (Jirovec and Templin, 2001).

The design of PV programs varies slightly, depending on the environment. The timing of prompts ranges from every 2 to 3 hours during waking hours. The program may include a verbal inquiry regarding the need to use the toilet, a physical check of the person to assess wetness, and assistance with mobility to access the toilet. The main goals of a PV program are to reduce the incidence of incontinent events, increase bladder awareness, and promote self-initiated toileting (Engberg et al., 2002).

A PV program can be directed at the individual or incorporated into the routine care of nursing-home residents. An individual program aims to identify the patient's normal pattern of toileting and coordinate a verbal prompt and assistance with toileting. The success of the individualized approach relies on a vigilant caregiver acting on nonverbal cues. A residential program may use set toileting times built into the residents' daily care schedule, and thus maintaining continence is more a matter of good timing than good training.

A recent Cochrane systematic review of nine studies comparing PV to normal care included 674 participants from the community and residential-care facilities. The authors concluded there was limited evidence that PV increased self-initiated voiding and decreased incontinence episodes. There was no evidence that the effects of the program are sustained over time or persist after stopping the program (Eustice et al., 2009). The literature also identified that PV programs were labor-intensive for caregivers and residential aged care staff. Several negative studies have listed reduced staff numbers, decreased staff motivation, and a lack of resources as the major barriers to the effective long-term implementation of PV programs (Pinkowski, 1996, Eustice et al., 2009). One study conducted by Ouslander and colleagues (2005) found a fourfold increase in labor costs associated with implementing PV programs compared with regular care.

In order to try to improve the outcome of PV programs, Schnelle et al. (2002) added incidental exercise to a PV program and compared it to routine patient care. Residents were randomized to control (normal care) or intervention (PV and exercise) groups. Each resident in the intervention group received 2-hourly toileting and a brief exercise session associated with the toileting. Dedicated research staff delivered the program from Monday to Friday for 8 hours a day over a period of 8 months. The exercise session was aimed at improving general strength, transfers, walking, and wheelchair ability. The intervention resulted in maintained or significantly improved physical performance outcome measures and a decreased frequency of episodes of incontinence in the intervention group compared with the placebo group. The study also recorded the time per resident required to carry out the program. The mean time for the intervention was 20 minutes, with 7 minutes for toileting, 3 minutes required to locate the resident, and 10 minutes to deliver the exercise program per episode of care. The entire intervention group showed a 100% improvement in mobility and distance walked, and a 44% improvement in appropriate toileting. Based on the study's time-management data, a finding was that one staff member per five residents is required to successfully implement the PV and exercise program. The authors acknowledge that a lack of resources is the main barrier to successfully implementing this type of program.

In community-dwelling older people, PV programs or individualized scheduling programs may be used by carers to manage continence, and are based on the same principles as the PV program in the residential-care setting. Family caregivers have the added advantage of understanding the daily habits of the person in their care and can tailor the toileting schedule to maximize success.

PV programs, however, are not designed to treat the cause of the incontinence but only to manage the problem. Whether the program is directed at community patients or residents in care, the predictors of success are cognitive ability, level of mobility, and the degree of support from a caregiver (Jirovec and Templin, 2001).

## Other interventions

Several other interventions for the prevention and management of incontinence have been reported in the literature, and have had varying degrees of success in older people with dementia. Pelvic floor exercises were seldom successful in a cognitively impaired population, owing to an inability to retain and follow instructions (Tobin and Brocklehurst, 1986).

## Medication use

Several case studies of medication usage were found in the literature linking incontinence to the use of cholinesterase inhibitors. The primary target for this class of drugs is the central nervous system, but such drugs are known to have systemic effects on the gastrointestinal tract and the bladder. Hashimoto et al. (2000) reported on 94 observed cases of donepezil use with a 7.4% incidence of incontinence in the first 2–14 days of treatment. They concluded that the findings strongly suggested a causal dose-dependent relationship between donepezil and incontinence. However, this has not been supported by findings from randomized controlled trials for donepezil or other cholinesterase inhibitors (Siegler and Reidenberg, 2004). The use of cholinesterase inhibitors may, in fact, have the opposite effect by improving cognitive ability and motivation in patients, resulting in lesser rates of incontinence (Sakakibara et al., 2008).

Detrusor hyperactivity or overactive bladder can be treated with antimuscarinic medication to improve continence. A small study by Lackner and colleagues (2008) of 50 women with dementia living in a nursing home compared the antimuscarinic drug oxybutynin to placebo for safety and tolerability. The researchers concluded that the study supported the use of 5 mg of oxybutynin in older female nursing-home residents with dementia and urge incontinence, as the treatment was well tolerated with little evidence of delirium or any short-term decline in cognition. The effect on UI was not reported.

Caution is advised when using medications to treat UI in this patient group owing to their anticholinergic effects. Older patients are generally particularly susceptible to drug-induced cognitive impairment due to age-related decreases in acetylcholine. The rapid decrease in acetylcholine activity produced by anti-cholinergic drugs in the brain of older patients can increase the risk of confusion, delirium, falls, disorientation, and memory impairment, and decrease levels of consciousness. Thus careful patient selection and monitoring is required if these drugs are concomitantly used in older patients, particularly in those older patients with dementia (Edwards and O'Connor, 2002, Kay et al., 2005).

## Continence aids

Both community-dwelling older people with dementia and those living in residential-care facilities generally use absorbent continence aids (e.g., pads or diapers). When worn by the individual they provide a means of managing incontinence, protecting clothing, and preserving dignity. The use of absorbent pads provides a level of social acceptability and security. On the negative side, the pads are bulky, may have an offensive odor, can lead to skin breakdown, and can make it very difficult to self-toilet. Residential care workers rely heavily on the use of pads to manage incontinence, and they are used more than PV programs because of time constraints. Wai and colleagues (2008) designed a novel pilot study to test a wireless system to detect wetness in incontinence pads to save staff time in manually monitoring residents. One resident was monitored for 1 week, with the system successfully detecting wetness 50% of the time compared with manual checks. Improvement in sensor placement and increased staff education may improve the outcome of future studies using this type of wireless technology.

The use of incontinence pads should not replace careful assessment and the review of treatable causes of incontinence (Pringle-Specht, 2005, Hägglund, 2010). When intractable UI is present, or as an end-of-life comfort measure, an indwelling catheter (IDC), either urethral or suprapubic, may be considered. Staff convenience is not a sufficient reason to initiate the long term use of IDCs, owing to the increased risk of urinary tract infections, urethral trauma, and patient discomfort.

## Caregiver burden

Successfully managing incontinence in an older person with dementia relies heavily on the support and diligence of the caregiver. The role of caregiver has been described as exhausting, difficult, and detrimental to the caregiver's own physical, psychological, and social well-being (Upton and Reed, 2005). The task of toileting can generate extra stress for caregivers and become the conduit for other challenging patient behaviors, such as resistance, aggression, and screaming and shouting. Studies indicate an increased caregiver burden is a major factor in the decision to institutionalize an individual with dementia (Upton and Reed, 2005). However, incontinence in isolation was not found to be a strong risk factor for nursing-home admission (Donaldson and Burns, 1999, Gaugler et al., 2009).

Staff working in residential aged care facilities have reported feelings of being frustrated and overwhelmed by the number of incontinent residents requiring assistance with toileting (Heine, 1986). Staff may often feel guilty about not adequately meeting the needs of all residents, and they find that the introduction of a PV program can create a conflict between the amount of work required for good patient care and the staff available (Yu and Kaltreider, 1987, Yu et al., 1991, O'Donnell et al., 1992, Durrant and Snape, 2003).

## Fecal incontinence

As previously mentioned, fecal incontinence is frequently underreported and causes considerable stress and embarrassment to the sufferer. It is estimated that the prevalence of fecal incontinence within the normal older population is between 2 and 5%, and may be considerably higher in the population of older people with dementia (Brocklehurst et al., 1999, Tarqid, 2007). A community-based study by Kalantar and colleagues (2002) found an overall prevalence rate of 11% among adults over 18 years. Prevalence rates in residential aged care facilities of up to 80% are noted in the literature (Ouslander et al., 1996, Brocklehurst et al., 1999, Chiang et al., 2000, Pringle-Specht, 2005, Tarqid 2007, Hägglund, 2010).

The risk factors associated with the development of fecal incontinence include cognitive impairment, decreased mobility, neurological diseases, stroke, irritable bowel syndrome, dehydration, poor diet, medications, inappropriate use of laxatives, and physical restraints (Brocklehurst et al., 1999, Ratnaike et al., 2000, Pringle-Specht, 2005, Leung and Rao, 2009). Management of the problem relies on treating the cause of the fecal incontinence. Constipation with overflow is routinely treated with laxatives and enemas in the first instance, followed by dietary modification such as increasing fluid and fiber intake and increasing exercise and physical activity.

Increased daily fiber intake has been shown to reduce fecal incontinence in a randomized controlled trial by Bliss and colleagues (2001), and scheduled toileting programs can also reduce the occurrence of fecal incontinence, as double incontinence occurs in 50 to 70% of incontinent older adults (Bliss et al., 2001, Tarqid, 2007). Other management tools include incontinence pads and the appropriate use of medication, such as antidiarrheal agents or laxatives.

## Recommendations

1. Undertake a comprehensive assessment to identify reversible and treatable causes of incontinence. Look particularly for urinary tract infection, constipation, and prostatic hypertrophy with secondary bladder hyperactivity.
2. Conduct a full review of current medication use, including over-the-counter laxative use, antipsychotics, and antidepressants.
3. Acknowledge caregiver stress and provide support and education on non-invasive cost-effective measures for managing incontinence, for example using protective sheeting on beds, sourcing a linen service, etc.
4. Implement individual incontinence management programs. Suggested components include:
   Allow adequate fluids during the day, and avoid fluids in the evening
   Ensure easy toilet access with grab rails, a toilet surround frame or raised toilet seat, and adequate lighting
   Ensure appropriate clothing with ease of access, for example using elasticized waistbands and Velcro closures rather than buttons or zips
   If pads are used, ensure they are easy to pull down so that toileting can be encouraged
   Follow a prompted toileting program with a fixed timing schedule
   Look for clues of a full bladder, including restlessness, pacing, pulling at pants
   Ensure appropriate mobility aids such as walking stick or frame are available to encourage independent mobility and access to toilet
   Consider medication or catheterization as a last resort.

---

### Case studies

Mrs. H is a 68-year-old woman who lives with her husband. She was diagnosed with AD 8 years ago, and her current MMSE score is 10/30. She remains physically mobile and socially appropriate. Mrs. H was independent in toileting and usually continent, and wore a light continence pad during the day. During a routine clinic visit Mr. H reported a new behavior that was causing him great distress. His wife had begun disposing of used continence pads and toilet paper in inappropriate places around the house, including cupboards and drawers. Strategies such as restricting Mrs. H to using one toilet in the house, removing all rubbish bins and other containers, locking cupboards where possible, and checking Mrs. H after toileting were partially effective for several months. Mrs. H then became more incontinent, and regular toileting every 2 hours with full assistance from Mr. H was started with reasonable success. Unfortunately Mrs H. became more aggressive and combative toward her husband, particularly during toileting, and she now needs to wear full continence pads 24 hours a day.

Mrs. Q is an 82-year-old woman with moderately severe dementia who resides in a dementia-specific residential-care facility. She has experienced worsening urinary incontinence for 2 years, which has been managed by regular toileting during the day and a full continence pad overnight. She has been becoming incontinent of feces over the past few months and has commenced wearing a continence pad during the day as well. She often removes this in inappropriate places, such as the dining room, and this has become a major behavioral issue, as she has a recent tendency to put her hand into the pad's contents and smear the feces around the room. Staff members have attempted to watch Mrs. Q and take her back to her room when she has opened her bowels but this has not always been successful. Consequently staff have designed an adhesive pad closure for Mrs. Q's pad that prevents her from removing it herself. Together with the use of a bulk laxative to ensure regular bowel motions, Mrs. Q's incontinence can be managed in such a way so as not to upset other residents.

---

**Key points**

- In dementia there is a loss of cognitive ability to interpret the sensation of a full bladder, loss of motivation to inhibit the passage of urine, and an inability to plan how to self-toilet. Together with dressing dyspraxia and visuospatial deficits, this leads to incontinence.
- Urinary incontinence occurs earlier in the course of vascular dementia, dementia with Lewy bodies, and frontotemporal dementia, than in Alzheimer's disease.

# References

Bliss, D., Jung, H., Savik, K., et al. (2001). Supplementation with dietary fibre improves faecal incontinence. *Nursing Research*, 50, 203–213.

Blok, B. Willemsen, T., Holstege, G. (1997). A PET study of brain control of micturition in humans. *Brain*, 120, 111–121.

Bravo, C. (2004). Urinary and faecal incontinence and dementia. *Reviews in Clinical Gerontology*, 14, 129–136.

Brocklehurst, J. (1993). Urinary incontinence in the community-analysis of a MORI poll. *British Medical Journal*. 306, 832–834.

Brocklehurst, J., Dickson, E., Windsor, J. (1999). Laxatives and faecal incontinence in long term care. *Nursing Standard*, 13, 32–36.

Chiang, L., Ouslander, J., Schnelle, J., et al. (2000). Dually incontinent nursing home residents: clinical characteristics and treatment differences. *Journal of the American Geriatrics Society*, 48, 673–676.

Davidson, H., Borrie, M., Crilly, R. (1991). Copy task performance and urinary incontinence in Alzheimer's disease. *Journal of the American Geriatrics Society*, 39, 467–471.

Del-Ser, T., Munoz, G., Hachinski, V. (1996). Temporal pattern of cognitive decline and incontinence is different in Alzheimer's disease and diffused Lewy body disease. *Neurology*, 46, 682–686.

Diehl-Schmid, J., Schulte-Overberg, J., Hartman, J., et al. (2007). Extrapyrmidal signs, primitive reflexes and incontinence in fronto-temporal dementia. *European Journal of Neurology*, 2007, 14, 860–864.

Donaldson, C., and Burns, A. (1999). Burden of Alzheimer's disease: Helping the patients and caregiver. *Journal of Geriatric Psychiatry and Neurology*. 12, 21–28.

Durrant, J. and Snape, J. (2003). Urinary incontinence in nursing homes for older people. *Age and Aging*, 32, 12–18.

Edwards, K. and O'Connor, J. (2002). Risk of delirium with concomitant use of tolterodine and acetycholinesterase inhibitors. *Journal of the American Geriatrics Society*, 50, 1165–1166.

Engberg, S., Sereika, S., McDowell, J., et al. (2002). Effectiveness of prompted voiding in treating urinary incontinence in cognitively impaired homebound older adults. *Journal of Wound, Ostomy and Continence Nurses Society*, 29, 252–265.

Eustice, S., Roe, B., Paterson, J. (2009). Prompted voiding for the management of urinary incontinence in adults. *The Cochrane Database of Systematic Reviews*, 2, CD002113.

Fowler, C., (2006). Integrated control of lower urinary tract – clinical perspective. *British Journal of Pharmacology*, 147, S14–S24.

Gaugler, J., Yu, F., Krichbaum, K., et al. (2009). Predictors of nursing home admission for persons with dementia. *Medical Care*, 47, 606.

Goode, P., Burgio, K., Richter, H., et al. (2010). Incontinence in older women. *Journal of the American Medical Association*, 303, 2172–2181.

Hägglund, D. (2010). A systematic literature review of incontinence care for persons with dementia: the research evidence. *Journal of Clinical Nursing*, 19, 303–312.

Hashimoto, M., Imamura, T., Tanimukai, S., et al. (2000). Urinary incontinence: an unrecognized adverse effect with Donepezil. *The Lancet*, 356, 568.

Heine, C. (1986). Burnout among nursing home personnel. *Journal of Gerontological Nursing*, 12, 14–18.

Hutchinson, S., Leger-Krall, S., Wilson, H. (1996). Toileting, a biobehavioral challenge in alzheimer's dementia care. *Journal of Gerontological Nursing*, 2, 18–27.

Jirovec, M., and Templin, T. (2001). Predicting success using individual scheduled toileting for memory impaired elders at home. *Research in Nursing & Health*, 24, 1–8.

Jirovec, M., and Wells, T. (1990). Urinary incontinence in nursing home residents with dementia: mobility- cognition paradigm. *Applied Nursing Research*, 3, 112–117.

Kalantar, J., Howell, S., Talley, N. (2002). Prevalence of faecal incontinence and associated risk factors. An underdiagnosed problem in the Australian community? *Medical Journal of Australia*, 176, 54–57.

Kay, G., Abou-Donia, M., Messer, W., et al. (2005). Antimuscarinic drugs for over-active bladder and their potential effects on cognitive function in older patients. *Journal of the American Geriatrics Society*, 53, 2195–2201.

Knight, M. (2000). Cognitive ability and functional status. *Journal of Advanced Nursing*, 31, 1459–1468.

Lackner, T., Wyman, J., McCarthy, T., et al. (2008). Randomised, placebo-controlled trial of the cognitive effect, safety and tolerability of oral extended release oxybutynin in cognitively impaired nursing home residents with urge urinary incontinence. *Journal of the American Geriatrics Society*, 56, 862–870.

Leung, F. and Rao, S. (2009). Faecal incontinence in the elderly. *Gastroenterology Clinics of North America*, 38, 503–511.

Miu, D., Lau, S., Szeto, S. (2010). Etiology and predictors of urinary incontinence and its effect on quality of life. *Geriatrics Gerontology International*, 10, 177–182.

O'Donnell, B., Drachman, D., Barnes. H., et al. (1992) Incontinence and trouble-some behaviours predict institutionalization in dementia. *Journal of Geriatric Psychiatry and Neurology*, 5, 45–52.

Ostbye, T., Seim, A., Krause, K., et al. (2004). A 10 year follow up study of urinary and faecal incontinence among the oldest old in the community: The Canadian study of health and aging. *Canadian Journal on Aging*, 23, 319–332.

Ouslander, J., Griffiths, P., McConnell, E., et al. (2005). Functional incidental training: randomised, controlled, crossover trial in veterans affairs nursing homes. *Journal of the American Geriatrics Society*, 53, 1091–1100.

Ouslander, J., Simmons, S., Schnelle, J., et al. (1996). Effects of prompted voiding on fecal continence among nursing home residents. *Journal of the American Geriatrics Society*, 44, 424–428.

Ouslander J., Zarit, S., Orr, N., et al. (1990). Incontinence among community dwelling dementia patients. Characteristics, management, and impact on caregivers. *Journal of the American Geriatrics Society*, 38, 440–444.

Pernezcky, R., Dieh-Schmid, J., Forstl, H., et al. (2008). Urinary incontinence and its functional anatomy in fronto temporal lobar degenerations. *European Journal of Nuclear Medical Molecular Imaging*, 35, 605–610.

Pinkowski, P.S. (1996). Prompted voiding in the long-term care facility. *Journal of Wound, Ostomy and Continence Nursing Society*, 23, 110–114.

Powell, M. and Rigby, D. (2002). Management of bowel dysfunction: evacuation difficulties. *Nursing Standard*, 14, 47–54.

Pringle-Specht, J. (2005). 9 myths of incontinence in older adults, *American Journal of Nursing*, 105, 58–68.

Pringle-Specht, J., Lyons, S., Maas, M. (2002). Patterns and treatments of urinary incontinence on special care units. *Journal of Gerontological Nursing*, 28, 13–21.

Ransmyr, G.N., Holliger, S., Schletterer, K., et al. (2008). Lower urinary track symptoms in dementia with Lewy bodies, Parkinson disease and Alzheimer's disease. *Neurology*, 70, 299–303.

Ratnaike, R., Milton, A., Olimpia, N. (2000). Drug associated diarrhoea and constipation in older people, *The Australian Journal of Hospital Pharmacy*, 30, 210–213.

Resnick, N. (1995). Urinary incontinence. *The Lancet*, 346, 94–99.

Sakakibara, R., Uchiyama, T., Yamanishi, T., et al. (2008). Dementia and lower urinary dysfunction: with a reference to anticholinergic use in elderly population. *The International Journal of Urology*, 15, 778–788.

Schnelle, J., Alessi, C., Simmons, S., et al. (2002). Translating research into practice: randomised controlled trial of exercise and incontinence care with nursing home residents. *Journal of the American Geriatrics Society*, 50, 1476–1483.

Siegler, E. and Reidenberg, M. (2004). Treatment of urinary incontinence with anticholinergics in patients taking cholinesterase inhibitors for dementia. *Clinical Pharmacology and Therapeutics*, 75, 484–488.

Tarqid, S. (2007). Faecal incontinence in older adults. *Clinics in Geriatric Medicine*, 23, 857–869.

Tobin, G.W. and Brocklehurst, J.C. (1986). The management of urinary incontinence in local authority residential homes for the elderly. *Age & Ageing*, 15, 292–298.

Upton, N. and Reed, V. (2005). The meaning of incontinence in dementia care. *The International Journal of Psychiatric Nursing Research*, 11, 1200–1210.

Wai, A., Fook, V., Jayachandran, M., et al. (2008). Smart wireless continence management system for persons with dementia. *Telemedicine and e-Health*, 14, 825–832.

Wilson, L. (2003). Continence and older people: the importance of functional assessment. *Nursing Older People*, 15, 22–28.

Wood, J. and Grafman, J. (2003). Human prefrontal cortex: processing and representational perspectives. *Nature Reviews, Neuroscience*, 4, 139–147.

Yap, P. and Tan, T. (2006). Urinary incontinence in dementia, a practical approach. *Australian Family Physician*, 35, 237–241.

Yu, L., Johnson, K., Kaltreider, D.L., et al. (1991). Urinary incontinence nursing home staff reaction toward residents. *Journal of Gerontological Nursing*, 17, 34–41.

Yu, L. and Kaltreider, D. (1987). Stressed nurses dealing with incontinent patients. *Journal of Gerontological Nursing*, 13, 27–30.

# 7

# Sleep disturbance

## Introduction

Age-related changes in sleep patterns are well documented in the older adult population. Changes occur in several areas, with increased time taken to fall asleep, more awakenings, and more time spent in the lighter stages of sleep. In addition, total sleep time, sleep efficiency, and rapid eye movement (REM)/non-rapid eye movement (NREM) cycles are reduced (Hornung et al., 2005, Cole and Richards, 2006, Fetveit and Bjorvatn, 2006).

In dementia, and particularly in Alzheimer's disease (AD), there is reduced sleep efficiency, increased amounts of NREM sleep, and an increase in the number of awakenings compared with age-matched controls (Gabelle and Dauvilliers, 2010). There is equally a comparative decrease in the amount of REM sleep, a reduction in total sleep length, and more sleep–wake rhythm disturbance (Chokroverty, 1996, Tractenberg et al., 2005a). The severity of these changes in sleep appears to increase concurrently with increasing dementia severity. Disrupted sleep patterns have a significant impact on patient and carer quality of life, with chronic sleep deprivation playing a key role in the decision to institutionalize the patient (Fetveit et al., 2003, McCurry et al., 2003, 2005, Howcroft and Jones, 2004, Cole and Richards, 2005, David et al., 2010). In diffuse Lewy body disease, REM sleep behavior disorder manifests as vivid and frightening dreams (Lee and Thomas, 2011).

Knowledge on the occurrence of sleep disorders in dementia has expanded over the last decade. The studies presented in this chapter confirm that sleep disturbance is a component of the behavioral symptomatology of dementia, with a detrimental impact on quality of life in both the person with dementia and their carer.

## Pathology of sleep disturbance

It is thought that changes that occur in circadian rhythm with advancing age are related to age-associated degenerative changes in the suprachiasmatic nucleus

(SCN) of the hypothalamus (Hornung et al., 2005, Craig et al., 2006, Van Dijk et al., 2006). Dementia can further change and disrupt the sleep–wake rhythm of the individual, as damage to the neural pathways interferes with the body's ability to initiate and maintain sleep. The pathology behind the marked changes in sleep patterns of AD patients is thought to be related to the presence of neurofibrillary tangles (but not amyloid plaques) within the SCN and the subsequent loss of neurons (Bliwise, 2004). This can explain the inversion of sleep rhythm and the day–night reversal that is seen in AD patients. The decrease in REM sleep is likely to be secondary to the degeneration and loss of cholinergic neurons in the nucleus basalis of Meynert and the loss of noradrenergic neurons in the brain stem (Chokroverty, 1996). It is probable that a combination of neuroanatomical and neurochemical changes associated with AD and other dementias all contribute to the disruption of the sleep–wake cycle (Harper et al., 2001, Obadinia et al., 2004, Bonanni et al., 2005, Dowling et al., 2005).

Recently disrupted sleep patterns have been suggested by Beaulieu-Bonneau and Hudon (2009) to be one of the core symptoms of mild cognitive impairment (MCI) in individuals who eventually develop dementia. A study of 65 community-dwelling MCI patients reported a high prevalence of movement-related sleep disorders, including restless leg syndrome and periodic leg movement. The current data on sleep disorders and MCI highlight two key questions: Are sleep disorders and cognitive impairment biomarkers for an underlying neurodegenerative disease, or do sleep disorders in fact contribute to the development of MCI (Bombois et al., 2010)?

## The epidemiology of sleep disorders in dementia

The association between dementia and sleep disorders is well documented in the literature, with between 25 and 50% of dementia patients reporting some sleep disturbance (Moran et al., 2005, Pandi-Perumal et al., 2005). Several large observational studies have identified patterns of sleep disturbance common to patients with dementia. The studies have assessed patients from the community, supported accommodation, and nursing-home care.

A study by Tractenberg et al. (2005a, 2005b) examined the sleep patterns of 263 community-dwelling dementia patients compared with a control group of 399 healthy older adults without dementia in the Oregon Brain Aging Study. The study found sleep problems were reported in the dementia participants with a significantly longer duration of disease and significantly lower scoring on function in activities of daily living. The study identified a range of sleep disturbances in both groups, with increased daytime sleep the most distinctive feature in the dementia group. These findings are supported by another study by Lee and colleagues (Lee, J.H., et al. 2007) who examined 137 community-dwelling dementia patients with a focus on the level of daytime sleepiness of the AD participants. The study found daytime sleepiness was associated with greater levels of impairment in functional status and a lower mean Mini-Mental State Examination (MMSE) score. Statistically significant results confirm a higher incidence of daytime sleepiness is associated with a lower MMSE, lower levels of functional capacity, and more clinically severe dementia. A number of other studies have also confirmed that increased daytime sleepiness and napping are frequently seen in dementia patients (Obadinia et al., 2004, Bonanni et al., 2005, Tractenberg et al., 2005b, Lee, J.H. et al., 2007, Rao et al., 2008, Rongve et al., 2010).

No association has been shown between the APOE-epsilon4 allele and an increased likelihood of developing sleep disturbance in people with AD (Craig et al., 2006). A small longitudinal study by Yesavage and colleagues (2003) also concluded that carrying the APOE-epsilon4 allele did not contribute to an increased likelihood of sleep disturbances. In fact, those participants who were APOE-epsilon4 negative showed a somewhat greater deterioration in sleep patterns over the 2.6 years of follow-up.

A number of smaller observational studies have used a combination of validated questionnaires, carer observation records, sleep diaries, biochemical measurements, and activity monitoring devices in assessment. These studies were conducted in a variety of settings including community, supported accommodation, and nursing-care facilities. The range of cognitive impairment varied greatly between care environments, with the majority of participants scoring below 15/30 on the MMSE. In separate studies by Gagnon and colleagues (2006), Cooke and colleagues (2006), and Bonanni and colleagues (2005), the "gold standard" of sleep assessment, polysomnography (Ancoli-Israel and Vittiello, 2006), was used to assess AD subjects in both laboratory and home settings. All studies reported disturbed sleep in the AD participants, with decreased REM sleep and decreased total sleep time. Cooke and colleagues (2006) performed home polysomnography on 76 people with AD who were currently taking the acetylcholinesterase inhibitors donepezil, galantamine, or rivastigmine. No differences in REM sleep were recorded between those patients on the different medications, but it was noted that the donepezil study group recorded a higher incidence of sleep architecture disturbances.

Several studies used a wrist-worn actigraph unit to monitor the activity of the AD patient over a period of time, frequently for 1 to 2 weeks. The units were worn 24 hours a day except when showering, and the data were analyzed by computer. These units are less invasive than polysomnography and are reliable in measuring sleep–wake parameters and rhythms over a longer period of time, which provides reliable and "naturalistic" data (Lee and Thomas, 2011). The studies identified several areas of dysfunction, including increases in sleep latency, daytime sleepiness, sleep arousals, sleep stage shifts and nocturnal awakenings, and a reduction in total sleep time, sleep efficiency, and REM/NREM cycles. A study by Hatfield and colleagues (2004) demonstrated that circadian dysfunction was a component of the behavioral symptomatology of dementia rather than an artifact of institutionalization.

Studies have consistently shown that those AD patients who resided in nursing homes with the lowest MMSE scores recorded the highest level of sleep disturbance. These results were attributed to the severity of dementia in the nursing-home population, environmental factors including poor lighting, institutional routines, and lower levels of daytime activity including exposure to sunlight (Ancoli-Israel et al., 1997, Sullivan and Richards 2004, Paavilainen et al., 2005, Fetveit and Bjorvatn, 2006).

## Intervention and treatment for sleep disturbance in dementia

### Light therapy

Exposure of the eyes to adequate light during the day can have a profound effect on the quality, duration, and timing of sleep. The retinohypothalamic tract mediates the effect of light on the circadian timing system, and the daily light–dark cycle is the primary synchronizer for the sleep–wake cycle (Dowling et al., 2005). The mechanism of action of the bright light on the circadian rhythm in dementia is not well understood, and studies have applied bright light therapy in the morning and evening with varying effects. The source, strength, and duration of the bright light varied between studies, and the majority of studies were carried out in high-level residential-care settings.

A review of 14 bright-light studies was performed by Kim et al. (2003). Each study considered dementia patients with sleep or behavioral disturbance, used bright light as an intervention, and reported changes in sleep and/or behavior. The review covered such areas as the season in which the treatment occurred, treatment time of day, dosage of bright light, patient behavior, sleep–wakefulness and circadian rhythm. The reported results from the studies were considered inconclusive because of the lack of control groups, blinded evaluations, and objective outcome measures, and the small sample sizes.

In the Cochrane systematic review of the effect of bright-light therapy on dementia by Forbes and colleagues (2009), 52 articles were retrieved. Following review only 5 met the inclusion criteria and only 3 were suitable for analysis. Patient compliance with the bright-light therapy and wearing the actigraph activity monitor were noted to be issues in the reviewed studies. The review concluded that there is little significant evidence of benefit for the effects of bright-light therapy on sleep, behavior, and mood disturbances associated with dementia.

In a slightly different use of light therapy, Fontana Gasio and colleagues (2003) reported a study of the effects of dawn/dusk simulation (DDS) light therapy on the circadian rhythm of 13 nursing-home patients. This observational study showed that DDS induced a shortening of sleep latency, a longer sleep duration, and less nocturnal activity.

### Medication

The use of sedating medication to improve sleep in patients with dementia should be considered with care (McCurry et al., 2007), as the side effects and risks associated with sedative-hypnotic medication may increase confusion or increase the risk of injury in this patient population (Richards et al., 2005).

Alternatives to sedative hypnotics have been studied, with melatonin considered in a number of studies. Melatonin is a pineal hormone that appears to be involved in the physiological regulation of sleep. It is secreted nocturnally and assists in the circadian regulation of sleep, as well as having significant sleep-promoting activity (Pandi-Perumal et al., 2005). In a study of melatonin use in 40 well older people, however, it was not shown to improve sleep (Baskett et al., 2003). In a study of 157 older people with dementia, Singer and colleagues (2003) randomized participants to three treatment arms: placebo; 2.5 mg slow-release melatonin; and 10 mg immediate-release melatonin. Wrist actigraphs were used to record data on sleep–wake cycles. Caregivers completed a daily sleep diary documenting patient bedtimes, lights-out time, and the time of melatonin administration. No statistically significant differences in objective sleep measures were seen between baseline and treatment periods for any of the three groups. Based on the collected actigraph data, melatonin was shown to be ineffective in this group of AD patients; however, there was a nonsignificant trend toward an improved duration of sleep in the 10 mg melatonin group.

Another long-term study of 189 residents in a group care facility combined melatonin with bright-light therapy. During the 3-year study, a modest benefit was found in the group randomized to the combined therapy. The authors recommend that melatonin be used in combination with light therapy in order to counteract any negative effects of melatonin on mood (Riemersma-van der Lek et al., 2008).

A systematic review of studies of melatonin treatment was conducted by de Jonghe and colleagues (2010). They reviewed four randomized controlled trials and five case studies, assessing a total of 330 patients. Mixed methodologies and various dose levels prevented any direct comparisons being drawn between the studies. The randomized trials reported less of an effect between the treatment and placebo groups than was reported in the case studies. This difference may be accounted for by the observational design and overestimation of the true effect in the case studies. Results from the case studies did suggest melatonin may have some effect in treating sundowning symptoms in dementia, and the authors recommended that further research was required in this area.

Duran and colleagues (2005) used risperidone (an atypical antipsychotic drug commonly used to treat the behavioral disturbances of dementia) in an open-label observational study to evaluate its effect on mood and behavior including sleep. Doses ranged from 0.25 mg twice daily to a maximum daily dose of 4 mg. The treatment was associated with a significant improvement in sleep–wake patterns, and the number of hours patients spent asleep at night was significantly increased from 5.5 at baseline to 7.1 at week 12. The study concluded that risperidone is associated with improvements in behavior and improvement in sleep-related disruption.

## Activity programs

Activity programs are a nonpharmacological approach to treating noctur-nal and daytime sleep disturbances in AD patients and are commonly used in residential care. Richards and colleagues (2005) designed an individualized social activity program for nursing-home patients. The study aimed to deliver an effective low-cost treatment to improve the sleep–wake patterns of the 139 participating patients with dementia. Individualized social activity interven-tions (ISAIs) were prepared by two certified therapeutic recreation specialists using four primary participant characteristics: interests, cognition, functional status, and napping patterns. Participants were randomly assigned to one of two groups: ISAI or usual-care control. The ISAI group received 1–2 hours of social activities in 15–30 minute sessions on 21 consecutive days between 9 am and 5 pm.The usual-care control group received normal care and participated in any scheduled activities that the nursing home provided. Results showed the ISAI group had significantly less daytime sleep, and daytime napping was reduced from 2 hours to 1.25 hours compared with the usual-care control group. In addition, the ratio of daytime to nighttime sleep had decreased in the activity group. However, the groups did not differ when measured on nighttime sleep quantity.

Eggermont et al. (2010) implemented a study in 19 nursing homes for patients with mild to moderate dementia, to measure the impact of 30 minutes of daily walking on nighttime restlessness. The treatment group received 30 minutes of supervised, self-paced walking daily, at a time convenient to the patient. The con-trol group received a social visit from a student. Each group wore an actigraph unit to monitor daytime and nighttime activity levels 1 week before the interven-tion, immediately following the intervention, and again 6 weeks post-study. The study failed to show any significant beneficial effect on nighttime restlessness. The authors suggest that the study results may have been influenced by the timing of the physical activity undertaken by the patients, as no standardized times were established in the protocol. Therefore while other research suggests that activity taken around 5–6 hours before bed is beneficial for rest, the intensity of the walk-ing activity and the amount of activity undertaken for the remainder of the day may have influenced the study outcome.

Community activity programs for AD patients with sleep disturbances rely on the motivation and cooperation of the carer for successful implementation. A study of 36 ambulatory community-dwelling AD patients by McCurry and col-leagues (2005) illustrated the importance of carer support in the implementation of a 6-week daily activity and sleep hygiene program with a 6-month follow-up period. The study showed improvements for patients in terms of length of sleep time, fewer night awakenings, and less time spent awake during the night in the intervention group. The authors concluded that daily walking, increased light exposure, and improved sleep hygiene measures were effective in improving sleep in people with dementia.

## Carer burden and sleep disturbance

Carer stress is reported as a key factor in the decision to institutionalize a care recipient. Sleep deprivation and frequent nocturnal awakenings add to the burden of caring for a person with dementia. However, a study by McCurry and colleagues (2007) highlighted the shortcomings inherent in basing patient sleep data solely on subjective carer reporting of sleep disturbances. In their study of 46 community AD patients, despite the carers reporting multiple sleep disturbances, 41% of patients in fact had actigraph sleep efficiencies within the normal range, and 43% averaged 8 or more hours of sleep nightly.

In a study by Creese and colleagues (2008) of 60 spousal caregivers of individuals with AD, carers reported having fair to poor sleep quality, with one-third reporting a decreased level of sleep quality over the previous year. The majority of carers attributed their disturbed sleep to their spouse's nocturnal behavior, and their self-reported physical and mental health were both significantly poorer than age-matched norms. Carers with poorer sleep quality and more frequent nocturnal disruptions had higher levels of depressive symptoms and role burden. A higher frequency of nocturnal disruptions also correlated with poorer carer mental health.

In order to reduce carer stress and worry about the nighttime activities of the person with dementia, Rowe and colleagues (2010) designed a study using electronic monitoring equipment. The 12-month study of 49 carers (24 treatment, 25 control) measured sleep patterns for 7 days over nine different time points. The study used a pre-test–post-test design to monitor sleep activity via actigraph, through questionnaires, and with the night monitoring system (NMS). The NMS contained elements of a home-security system with the inclusion of bed sensors and movement detectors. The carers were alerted to any movement via text, alarm, and voice through a keypad next to their bed. Despite the monitoring, the study authors reported no significant improvement in the carers' stress or worry levels compared with the control group. Explaining these results is the NMS, alerting some carers to activity they would have previously slept through and hence disturbing them more during the night. In future the planned addition of "smart" features will allow patterns of safe activity to be programmed into the system, reducing the number of alerts for the carer.

The provision of residential respite care to reduce carer burden is often central to the support of AD patients and carers in the community. Lee, D. et al. (2007) examined the effects of 2 weeks' residential respite care on the sleep patterns of carers and people with AD. Primary sleep outcomes were derived for the people with dementia and the carers from 6 weeks of continuous wrist actigraph measurements, including 2 weeks baseline, 2 weeks during the residential respite care, and 2 weeks follow-up. For carers, respite periods were associated with a significant increase in total sleep time per night and total time spent in bed at night, and improvements in subjective sleep quality. For patients, however, respite was associated with significant increases in sleep-onset latency, reductions in total sleep time per night, and weakening of the circadian activity rhythm. This study confirms the transition from respite care back to the home environment can be difficult for people with dementia and their carers.

## Recommendations

1. Inquire about sleep disturbances for all patients presenting with cognitive impairment and dementia, including reviewing patient sleep habits with the caregiver, to ensure the recognition and management of sleep disorders in this population.
2. Conduct a full physical review of the patient, including the assessment and treatment of any pain.
3. Ensure that factors that may disturb sleep have been assessed and managed, for example current medication, pain, heat, cold, and infection.
4. Encourage good sleep hygiene measures by keeping noise to a minimum, keeping the room dark, and maintaining a comfortable temperature. Discourage daytime napping and engage the person with dementia in regular physical activities. Maintain regular sleep–wake routines and meal schedules and limit caffeine intake, restricting this after 2.30 pm.
5. Consider implementing a scheduled routine of daily physical exercise and increase the amount of exposure to daylight.
6. Choose nonpharmaceutical treatment options over pharmaceutical interventions before considering the use of sedative medication to manage sleep disturbance, and then only use melatonin and sedating medications with caution in this patient group.

## Case studies

Mr. J is an 81-year-old man with moderately severe AD. He had been cared for by his wife for many years with gradually increasing care needs. He fell in the shower one morning and sustained a fractured pelvis. He was admitted to hospital and after several weeks of attempting to regain mobility he was considered to require nursing-home placement. After his arrival in the nursing home he was found to be awake and quite noisy at night, and drowsy and sleeping most of the day. Sedative medication in the evening did not seem to have any effect and he remained disruptive and difficult to manage during the night. His general practitioner and the nursing-home staff met with Mr. J's wife and family and a care plan was developed. Family members agreed to spend most of the day with Mr. J, keeping him active and awake. In the evening he was given paracetamol for possible discomfort, and slow-release melatonin (2 mg) was administered. No other sedation was used. Over 2 weeks his sleep patterns changed and Mr. J was able to remain awake for most of the day, with just a short nap after the midday meal, later sleeping from about 10 pm to 5 am most nights. The melatonin was withdrawn after approximately 2 months but he remains on regular paracetamol in the evenings.

Mrs. Y is a 58-year-old woman who lives with her two sons in her own home. She had a diagnosis of MCI made 2 years ago after presenting to the memory clinic with short-term memory problems and difficulty sleeping. Her slightly impaired memory function has remained stable but her sleep is broken and she rarely sleeps more than 5 hours each night. She says she worries about her memory, and how she will cope. She has been given advice about sleep hygiene measures, and has begun walking for an hour each afternoon. She has also been commenced on an antidepressant, as she had a number of depressive symptoms. Her sleep pattern has improved and she is now sleeping for between 6 and 7 hours each night, without needing to use night sedation. She has learned relaxation techniques for use if she has problems falling asleep or wakes during the night, and finds these useful and effective.

### Key points

- Changes in sleep occur in many older people, but are more prominent in people with dementia, particularly Alzheimer's disease, with up to 50% reporting significant sleep disturbance.
- The circadian rhythm is disrupted in Alzheimer's disease, with delays and fragmentation of the sleep–wake cycle, and increased nighttime wakenings and increased daytime sleeping.
- The severity of sleep disturbance increases with the severity of the dementia.

## References

Ancoli-Israel, S., Klauber, M.R., Jones, D.W., et al. (1997). Variations in circadian rhythms of activity, sleep, and light exposure related to dementia in nursing-home patients. *Sleep*, 20, 18–23.

Ancoli-Israel, S. and Vittiello, M. (2006). Sleep in dementia. *American Journal of Geriatric Psychiatry*, 14, 91–94.

Baskett, J.J, Broad, J.B., Wood, P.C., et al. (2003). Does melatonin improve sleep in older people? A randomised crossover trial, *Age and Ageing*, 32, 164–170.

Beaulieu-Bonneau, S. and Hudon, C. (2009). Sleep disturbances in older adults with mild cognitive impairment. *International Psychogeriatrics*, 21, 645–666.

Bliwise, D.L. (2004). Sleep disorders in Alzheimer's disease and other dementias. *Clinical Cornerstone*, 6, S16–28.

Bombois, S., Derambure, P., Pasquier, F., et al. (2010). Sleep disorders in aging and dementia. *Journal of Nutrition, Health & Aging*, 14, 212–217.

Bonanni, E., Maestri, M., Tognoni, G. et al. (2005). Daytime sleepiness in mild and moderate alzheimer's disease and its relationship with cognitive impairment, *Journal of Sleep Research*, 14, 311–317.

Chokroverty, S. (1996). Sleep and degenerative neurologic disorders. *Neurologic Clinics*, 14, 807–827.

Cole, C. and Richards, K. (2005). Sleep and cognition in people with Alzheimer's disease. *Issues in Mental Health Nursing*, 26, 687–698.

Cole, C. and Richards, K. (2006). Sleep in persons with dementia: Increasing quality of life by managing sleep disorders. *Journal of Gerontological Nursing*, 32, 48–53.

Cooke, J. R., Loredo, J.S., Liu, L., et al. (2006). Acetycholinesterase inhibitors and sleep architecture in patients with Alzheimer's disease. *Drugs and Aging*, 23, 503–511.

Craig, D., Hart, D., Passmore, A. (2006). Genetically increased risk of sleep disruption in Alzheimer's disease. *Sleep*, 29, 1003–1007.

Creese, J., Bedard, M., Brazil, K., et al. (2008). Sleep disturbances in spousal caregivers of individuals with Alzheimer's disease. *International Psychogeriatrics*, 20,149–161.

David, R., Zeitzer, J., Friedman, L., et al. (2010). Non pharmacological management of sleep disturbance in Alzheimer's disease. *The Journal of Nutrition, Health & Aging*, 14, 203–206.

De Jonghe, A., Korevaar, J., Van Muster, B., et al. (2010). Effectiveness of melatonin treatment on circadian rhythm disturbances in dementia. Are there implications for delirium? A systematic review. *International Journal of Geriatric Psychiatry*, 25, 1201–1208.

Dowling, G.A., Hubbard, E. M., Mastick, J., et al. (2005). Effect of morning bright light treatment for rest-activity disruption in institutionalized patients with severe Alzheimer's disease. *International Psychogeriatrics*, 17, 221–236.

Duran, J., Greenspan, A., Diago, J.I., et al. (2005). Evaluation of risperidone in the treatment of behavioural and psychological symptoms and sleep disturbances associated with dementia. *International Psychogeriatrics*, 17, 591–604.

Eggermont, L., Blankvoort, C., Scherder, E. (2010). Walking and night-time restlessness in mild-to-moderate dementia: a randomized controlled trial. *Age and Aging*, 39, 746–761.

Fetveit, A. and Bjorvatn, B. (2006). Sleep duration during the 24-hour day is associated with the severity of dementia in nursing home patients. *International Journal of Geriatric Psychiatry*, 21, 945–950.

Fetveit, A., Skjerve, A., Bjorvatn, B. (2003). Bright light treatment improves sleep in institutionalized elderly-an open trial. *International Journal of Geriatric Psychiatry*, 18, 520–526.

Fontana Gasio, P., Krauchi, K., Cajochen, C., et al. (2003). Dawn-dusk simulation light therapy of disturbed circadian rest-activity cycles in demented elderly. *Experimental Gerontology*, 38, 207–216.

Forbes, D., Morgan, D.G., Bangma, J., et al. (2009). Light therapy for managing sleep, behaviour, and mood disturbances in dementia (review). *The Cochrane Library*, 4. Available at: http://onlinelibrary.wiley.com/doi/10.1002/14651858. CD003946.pub3/pdf [Accessed February 15, 2012].

Gabelle, A. and Dauvilliers, Y. (2010). Sleep and dementia, *The Journal of Nutrition, Health & Aging*, 14, 201–202.

Gagnon, J, F., Petit, D., Fantini, M.L., et al. (2006). REM sleep behaviour disorder and REM sleep without atonia in probable Alzheimer's disease, *Sleep*, 29, 1321–1325.

Harper, D.G., Stopa, E.G., McKee, A.C., et al.(2001). Differential circadian rhythm disturbances in men with Alzheimer's disease and frontotemporal degeneration, *Archives of General Psychiatry*, 58, 353–360.

Hatfield, C.F., Herbert, J., van Someren, E.J., et al. (2004). Disrupted daily activity/rest cycles in relation to daily cortisol rhythms of home-dwelling patients with early Alzheimer's dementia. *Brain*, 127, 1061–1074.

Hornung, P., Danker-Hopfe, H., Heuser, I. (2005). Age-related changes in sleep and memory: Commonalities and interrelationships. *Experimental Gerontology*, 40, 279–285.

Howcroft, D. and Jones, R. (2004). Does modafinil have the potential to improve disrupted sleep patterns in patients with dementia? *International Journal of Geriatric Psychiatry*, 20, 492–495.

Kim, S., Song, H., Yoo, S. (2003). The effect of bright light on sleep and behaviour in dementia: An analytic review, *Geriatric Nursing*, 24, 239–243.

Lee, D., Morgan, K., Lindesay, J. (2007). Effect of institutional respite care on the sleep of people with dementia and their primary caregiver. *Journal of the American Geriatrics Society*, 55, 252–258.

Lee, D. and Thomas, A. (2011). Sleep in dementia and caregiving- assessment and treatment implications: A review. *International Psychogeriatrics*, 23, 190–201.

Lee, J.H., Bliwise, D.L., Ansari, F.P., et al. (2007). Daytime sleepiness and functional impairment in Alzheimer's disease. *The American Journal of Geriatric Psychiatry*, 15, 620–626.

McCurry, S., Gibbons, L.E., Logsdon, R.G., et al. (2003). Training caregivers to change the sleep hygiene practices of patients with dementia: the NITE-AD project. *Journal of the American Geriatrics Society*, 51, 1455–1460.

McCurry, S. Gibbons, L.E., Logsdon, R.G., et al. (2005). Nighttime insomnia treatment and education for Alzheimer's disease: a randomized, controlled trial. *Journal of the American Geriatrics Society*, 53, 793–802.

McCurry, S., Gibbons, L.E., Logsdon, R.G., et al. (2007). Factors associated with caregiver reports of sleep disturbances in persons with dementia. *The American Journal of Geriatric Psychiatry*, 14, 112–120.

Moran, M., Lynch., C.A., Walsh, C. et al. (2005). Sleep disturbance in mild to moderate Alzheimer's disease, *Sleep Medicine*, 6, 347–352.

Obadinia, S., Noroozian, M., Shahsavand, S., et al. (2004). Evaluation of insomnia and daytime napping in Iranian Alzheimer's disease patients. *The American Journal of Geriatric Psychiatry*, 12, 517–522.

Paavilainen, P., Korhonen, I., Lotjonen, J., et al. (2005). Circadian activity rhythm in demented and non-demented nursing home residents measured by telemetric actigraphy. *Journal of Sleep Research*, 14, 61–68.

Pandi-Perumal, S., Zisapel, N., Srinivasn, V., et al. (2005). Melatonin and sleep in aging population, *Experimental Gerontology*, 40, 911–925.

Rao, V. Spiro, J., Samus, Q.M., et al. (2008). Insomnia and daytime sleepiness in people with dementia residing in assisted living: findings from the Maryland Assisted Living Study. *International Journal of Geriatric Psychiatry*, 23, 199–206.

Richards, K., Beck, C., O'Sullivan, P., et al. (2005). Effect of individual social activity on sleep in nursing home residents with dementia. *Journal of the American Geriatrics Society*, 53, 1510–1517.

Riemersma-van der Lek, R., Swaab, D., Twisk, J., et al. (2008). Effect of bright light and melatonin on cognitive and noncognitive function in elderly residents of group care facility. *Journal of the American Medical Association*, 299, 2642–2655.

Rongve, A., Boeve, B., Aarsland, D. (2010). Frequency and correlates of caregiver-reported sleep disturbances in a sample of persons with early dementia, *Journal of the American Geriatrics Society*, 58, 480–486.

Rowe, M., Kairalla, J., McCrae, C. (2010). Sleep in dementia caregivers and the effect of a night time monitoring system. *Journal of Nursing Scholarship*, 42, 338–347.

Singer, C., Tractenberg, R.E., Kaye, J., et al. (2003). A multicenter, placebo-controlled trial of melatonin for sleep disturbances in Alzheimer's disease, *Sleep*, 26, 893–901.

Sullivan, S. and Richards, K. (2004). Predictions of circadian sleep-wake rhythm maintenance in elders with dementia. *Aging & Mental Health*, 8, 143–152.

Tractenberg, R., Singer, C., Kaye, J. (2005a). Characterizing sleep problems in persons with Alzheimer's disease and normal elderly. *Journal of Sleep Research*, 15, 97–103.

Tractenberg, R., Singer, C., Kaye, J. (2005b). Symptoms of sleep disturbance in persons with Alzheimer's disease and normal elderly. *Journal of Sleep Research*, 14, 177–185.

Van Dijk, K., Lijpen, M.W., Van Someren, E.J., et al. (2006). Peripheral electrical nerve stimulation and rest-activity rhythm in Alzheimer's disease. *Journal of Sleep Research*, 15, 415–423.

Yesavage, J., Friedman, L., Kraemer, H., et al. (2003). Sleep/wake disruption in Alzheimer's disease: APOE status and longitudinal course. *Journal of Geriatric Psychiatry and Neurology*, 17, 20–24.

# 8

# Visual dysfunction

## Introduction

Visual dysfunction refers to restrictions in visual function, and there is a substantial body of research that identifies that visual dysfunction occurs in Alzheimer's disease (AD) and many of the other dementias. Patients may present with complaints of visual problems early in the disease process, well before problems with memory are identified. Altered contrast sensitivity and visual acuity, particularly in conditions of low light, as well as changes in the patient's color vision, can impact upon activities of daily living (ADL) for individuals with dementia. Impaired visual acuity may also be linked to increased occurrence of visual hallucinations. Visual field defects, resulting in loss of part of the field of vision, and problems with visuospatial perception, leading to difficulty with depth perception, are also known to occur.

Visual dysfunction in dementia may underlie many of the difficulties experienced by patients in undertaking their ADLs. Some of the common visual symptoms identified by patients and carers for which an ophthalmologist consultation is sought include blurred and distorted vision, difficulty reading and writing, problems with depth perception and bumping into objects, and difficulty identifying or locating familiar objects or people, driving a car, walking outdoors, manipulating objects, dressing, or judging distances (Mancil, 1994, Geldmacher, 2003, Lee and Martin, 2004). No studies have identified the prevalence of visual dysfunction in dementia, and most information is from case reports, case–control studies and cohort studies, and these most commonly relate to AD.

## Pathology of visual dysfunction in dementia

The underlying pathophysiology of visual dysfunction in AD and other dementias remains unclear, with studies suggesting a number of different causes. This may reflect the clinical variation seen in AD, and individual differences in disease progression, as well as different research methodologies (Nobili and Sannita, 1997). Neuroimaging and neuropathological studies have provided much of the information relating to the pathophysiology of visual dysfunction. Two investigative techniques, confocal scanning laser ophthalmoscopy (CSLO) (to view the optic nerve fiber layer), and optical coherence tomography (OCT) (to measure the thickness of the peripapillary retinal nerve fiber layer) are noninvasive imaging techniques for identifying underlying pathology in dementia-related visual dysfunction (Danesh-Meyer et al., 2006, Iseri et al., 2006).

There is a substantial body of research that ties visual impairment to underlying cortical damage (Morrison et al., 1991, Mielke et al., 1995, Armstrong, 1996, Hof et al., 1997, Giannakopoulos et al., 1999, Boxer et al., 2003). Both Mendez and colleagues (Mendez et al., 1990) and Cronin-Golomb (1995) have suggested that the visual defects in dementia are more likely to be related to pathological changes in the primary visual and association cortices in dementia than to changes in the retina or optic nerve. Deficits in the parietal and occipital cortices, including the primary visual cortex, have also been identified by Pietrini and colleagues (Pietrini et al., 1996).

However, a number of researchers have identified neurodegenerative changes in the retina and optic nerve in AD and other dementias (Blanks et al., 1991). Retinal nerve fiber layer (RNFL) thickness has been found to be significantly reduced in patients with mild cognitive impairment (MCI) and dementia compared with controls, using OCT of the retina. Paquet and colleagues examined 49 patients with MCI or dementia and 15 healthy controls, and found similar reductions in RNFL thickness in both MCI patients and mild dementia patients. They suggest that the RNFL is involved early during the course of amnestic MCI and dementia (Paquet et al., 2007).

A study by Iseri and colleagues (2006) demonstrated a reduction in the thickness of the parapapillary and macular retinal nerve fiber layer, and reduced macular volume in patients with dementia, using OCT. The reduction in macular volume was associated with the severity of cognitive impairment. Pham and colleagues (2006) identified a significant, cross-sectional association between late age-related macular degeneration (AMD) and cognitive impairment in a large study of 3500 older people. Cognitive impairment was found in 18% of people with late AMD and 8.4% with early AMD, compared with 2.6% in people without AMD. The association was weaker but remained significant after excluding vision-related items from the Mini-Mental State Examination (MMSE) (Pham et al., 2006).

Optic nerve changes in AD have been identified in both recent research (Danesh-Meyer et al., 2006, Paquet et al., 2007) and older studies (Hinton et al., 1986). In a small study of nine patients with AD and eight age-matched controls, Berisha and colleagues identified quantifiable retinal abnormalities in early dementia with a specific pattern of retinal nerve fiber layer loss, narrowing of veins, and decreased retinal blood flow, and concluded that there was evidence suggesting that visual disturbances in patients with dementia were due to pathologic changes in the retina and optic nerve, as well as to higher cortical impairment (Berisha et al., 2007).

An imaging study by Koronyo-Hamaoui and colleagues (2011) examined the brains and retinas of eight patients with AD confirmed at postmortem and those of five suspected AD patients. The imaging study confirmed the presence of amyloid plaques in the retinas, and the authors suggest that the finding may provide a specific diagnostic biomarker for the detection of early AD. As well as changes to the retina and optic nerve, one study has identified beta-amyloid in the cytosol of cells in the lens of patients with AD (Goldstein et al., 2003).

## The impact of visual dysfunction in people with dementia

The impact of dementia-associated visual dysfunction on the person with dementia can be considerable (Mendez et al., 1990, Cronin-Golomb et al., 1991, 1995, Cronin-Golomb, 1995, Trick et al., 1995, Baker et al., 1997, Rizzo et al., 2000, Lee and Martin, 2004, Fernandez et al., 2007). Patients may present with visual symptoms before the development of other signs of dementia. These include blurred or distorted vision, difficulties with reading, loss of part of the field of vision, prominent visuospatial problems, inability to recognize faces or familiar objects, and environmental disorientation. These symptoms are sometimes considered to be part of the visual variant of AD (VVAD), which has gained recognition in the past 10 years (Geldmacher, 2003, Lee and Martin, 2004).

Other dementias may also present with visual problems. Posterior cortical atrophy is associated with prominent visual deficits (Benson et al., 1988, Victoroff et al., 1994, Hof et al., 1997, Mendez et al., 2002, Schmidtke et al., 2005). Visual hallucinations are a hallmark feature of dementia with Lewy bodies, and visuospatial impairments may also be present early in the disease (Collerton et al., 2003). Significant visual dysfunction may also be a feature of many of the less common dementias such as Creutzfeldt–Jakob disease (CJD) (de Seze et al., 1998, Cooper et al., 2005) and cerebral autosomal dominant arteriopathy with subcortical infarcts and leukoencephalopathy (CADASIL) (Cumurciuc et al., 2004, Ravaglia et al., 2004). However, even patients who do not present with visual symptoms as part of their dementia have been shown to experience visual dysfunction when tested (Rizzo et al., 2000).

## Features of visual dysfunction in dementia

### Contrast sensitivity

**Contrast sensitivity** refers to the ability to distinguish objects from their background. Contrast sensitivity measures are highly sensitive to alterations in the visual system, and there is strong evidence that dementia, particularly AD, affects contrast sensitivity. The majority of studies conducted into contrast sensitivity for patients with dementia have identified impairments (Cronin-Golomb et al., 1991, 1995, Gilmore and Levy, 1991, Rizzo et al., 1992, Bassi et al., 1993, Hutton et al.,

1993, Gilmore and Whitehouse, 1995, Mendola et al., 1995, Keri et al., 1999, Rizzo et al., 2000, Fernandez et al., 2007). Cormack and colleagues summarized a range of research results and discussed the potential impact of a loss of contrast sensitivity on ADL and navigational ability, which may also affect the risk of falls. They recommend strategies to reduce the ADL and behavioral impact of contrast sensitivity deficits. Strategies could include both the correction of conditions that may additionally impact contrast sensitivity and visual acuity, such as cataracts, and environmental changes, such as improving lighting and the use of high-contrast markers (Cormack et al., 2000).

## Visual acuity

**Visual acuity** refers to the ability to see objects clearly and accurately both near and in the distance. Most eye test charts are designed as a measure of visual acuity. Lakshiminarayan and colleagues reported that dementia patients, including those with vascular dementia and AD, showed decreased visual acuity compared with normal controls (Lakshminarayanan et al., 1996). The 1993 study by Bassi and colleagues reported that patients with dementia had significantly poorer visual acuity than cognitively normal controls (Bassi et al., 1993). However, some studies have not found changes in visual acuity in patients with dementia significantly greater than those of normal aging (Katz and Rimmer, 1989, Mendez et al., 1990, Cronin-Golomb et al., 1991, Rizzo et al., 2000). Cormack suggests that this may be owing to the fact that measures of visual acuity are commonly taken in conditions of ideal luminance and contrast, which do not reflect the visual conditions in day-to-day life, and may therefore fail to reflect the real problems experienced in visual acuity by patients with dementia (Cormack et al., 2000).

Results from a large study of more than 3500 older people showed a significant association between impaired visual acuity and cognitive impairment (MMSE<24). After adjusting for age, sex, education, and history of stroke, people with vision impairment had a lower mean MMSE score than those with normal vision, regardless of whether vision-related items were included or excluded. People with probable cognitive impairment also had lower mean visual acuity than those without. The authors suggest that age-related decline and the effect of visual impairment on the measurement of cognition only partly explain the association between sensory and cognitive impairments in older people (Tay et al., 2006). The Leiden 85-Plus Study of 590 very old people also found both hearing and vision impairment were associated with lower scores on the MMSE, and that visual impairment was further associated with poorer scores on memory and cognitive speed (Gussekloo et al., 2005).

## Visual fields

**Visual field** refers to the amount of the environment seen by each eye, when both eyes are looking forward. Numerous case reports document the impact of AD and the other dementias on visual fields (Mancil, 1994, Brazis et al., 2000), and a number of studies have found that dementia may be associated with visual field defects such as an homonymous hemianopia (loss of half the field of vision in each eye) without any corresponding deficits on neuroimaging (Mendez et al., 1990, Lee and Martin, 2004). In a 1995 study, Trick and colleagues (1995) examined the visual fields of 61 patients with dementia and 61 subjects without dementia, using perimetry to detect the ability to see a light flash in different parts of the visual field. They reported that visual sensitivity (ability to see the light flash) was reduced in patients with dementia throughout the visual field, and most pronounced in the lower visual field. Patients with more severe dementia exhibited greater reductions in visual sensitivity. On follow-up, 60% of dementia patients demonstrated progression of visual field loss (Trick et al., 1995). Visual field deficits have also been found as early symptoms in CJD (Kropp et al., 1999, Brazis et al., 2000, Cooper et al., 2005).

## Visuospatial dysfunction

**Visuospatial function** refers to the ability to perceive visually the spatial relationships between objects, and remain visually orientated in space. This function allows the individual to navigate through the physical environment, locate and manipulate objects, and carry out basic and instrumental ADL. There is a considerable body of evidence indicating that dementia is associated with visuospatial dysfunction (Mendez et al., 1990, 1997, Fujimori et al., 1997, Tetewsky and Duffy, 1999, Rizzo et al. 2000, Lee and Martin, 2004). In 1995, Kaskie and Storandt examined visuospatial impairment in 125 individuals with mild dementia and compared them with 146 individuals without dementia, concluding that visuospatial deficit was apparent even in very mild AD (Kaskie and Storandt, 1995).

It has been suggested that visuospatial difficulties may underlie a number of problems with ADL for patients with dementia, including difficulty dressing, misreaching for objects, bumping into objects, misjudging steps or uneven surfaces, and losing their way in a familiar environment (Mancil, 1994).

Butter and colleagues suggest that visual symptoms in AD are related primarily to visuospatial deficits. They tested 14 patients with AD who had visual symptoms prominent enough to prompt ophthalmologic consultation compared with 11 patients with AD who lacked such visual symptoms, and a control group of 53 subjects without AD. Relative to controls, both groups of patients with dementia performed poorly on all visual tests. Patients with AD who had prominent visual symptoms differed significantly from those without prominent visual symptoms only in their relatively poor visuospatial test scores (Butter et al., 1996).

## Other visual symptoms

In a study of 30 AD patients in the community compared with 30 controls, Mendez and colleagues (1990) found that visual symptoms occurred in 43% of patients, and were particularly related to disturbances in spatial localization and object recognition. The inability to search for and find an object in the visual environment, and difficulty reaching for objects, were described in many of the patients. More than half the patients had difficulties visually recognizing simple objects such as a book, a house, a boat, or a cup, and also had difficulty recognizing pictures of famous people. Those with the more severe cognitive deficits had the most complex visual disturbances (Mendez et al., 1990).

In 1997, Mendez and colleagues investigated hemispatial neglect in 15 patients with mild to moderate AD, compared with 15 matched controls, on four measures of neglect. The group with AD was significantly impaired in attending to left hemispace, and Mendez suggested that future investigations might implicate neglect in visually related deficits of dementia, such as the difficulty with left turns when driving (Mendez et al., 1997). Impaired performance in visual tests was correlated with cognitive impairment in a study conducted by Rizzo and associates. The 43 patients in the AD group had impairments in visuospatial construction, higher visual perception and memory and processing of complex motion, and more than twice the loss of "useful field of view" compared with the 22 controls. Useful field of view size decreased in conjunction with overall cognitive decline (Rizzo et al., 2000).

Optic flow is the visual motion seen as a result of the observer's own movements. Tetewsky and Duffy (1999) suggest that impaired optic flow perception in AD may interfere with the use of visual information to guide self-movement and maintain spatial orientation. They studied optic flow in 22 AD patients and identified impaired ability to see optic flow in half of the patients, compared with both elderly and young controls. They found an association between impaired optic flow perception and poor performance on a spatial navigation test (Tetewsky and Duffy, 1999).

Impairments in color vision have been noted in some studies of people with AD, and Pache and colleagues (2003) examined the performance of 26 patients with AD compared with 25 controls on standardized tests of color vision. They used the Ishihara color vision test and also a test designed for children to avoid problems due to cognitive deficits. They found a significant difference in color vision between the two groups, with clear deficiencies in color vision in the group with AD compared with controls (Pache et al., 2003).

## Hallucinations

The impact of impaired visual function on the occurrence of visual hallucinations in dementia has been the subject of some research (McShane et al., 1995, Devos et al., 2005). In 1999, Chapman and colleagues investigated the link between impaired visual acuity and hallucinations in patients with dementia. They investigated visual acuity in 50 patients with probable dementia and found that impaired visual acuity and the severity of cognitive impairments were significantly associated with visual hallucinations. Visual acuity was significantly more impaired in patients with hallucinations and no patients with hallucinations had normal acuity (Chapman et al., 1999). Holroyd and colleagues screened 98 patients with AD and found that 18% of patients with AD experienced visual hallucinations. The authors report that older age, lower visual acuity in the "best eye," and visual agnosia correctly classified 91% of patients as hallucinators versus non-hallucinators

(Holroyd and Sheldon-Keller, 1995). Murgatroyd and Prettyman compared 30 patients with dementia who had experienced hallucinations with 30 dementia patients who had not, and found that half of the patients experiencing hallucinations had very poor visual acuity (Murgatroyd and Prettyman, 2001). On the basis of a control group comparison study, Pliskin and colleagues propose that isolated visual hallucinations in the older adult may be an indication of the early stages of dementia. They identified neuropsychological changes commonly associated with the early stages of dementia in their case series of 15 patients with visual hallucinations (Pliskin et al., 1996).

## Vision issues in residential-care facilities

In a retrospective cohort study in 2005, Koch and colleagues (2005) reviewed the prevalence of uncorrected visual disorders in 85 nursing-home patients with dementia. Over 94% of patients required glasses for the correction of presbyopia, myopia, or both. Of those who required glasses, more than 31% had not been using them since entering the nursing home. Some residents were too cognitively impaired to request their glasses, others had broken or misplaced them, and some had prescriptions that were no longer sufficient to correct their vision. The authors made three recommendations intended to improve visual acuity in nursing-home residents with dementia: (1) label eyewear in appropriate patient populations to provide rapid identification in the event of misplacement; (2) ensure that an extra pair of glasses be made available in the event of loss or damage; and (3) ensure that all residents have annual or biannual eye tests (Koch et al., 2005).

In 2004, an expert nursing-home panel review identified 13 quality indicators related to vision impairment relevant to residential care. These included providing annual eye examinations for residents, ensuring access to corrective lenses, offering cataract surgery where appropriate, and updating lens prescriptions as needed (Saliba et al., 2004).

## Management of visual dysfunction in people with dementia

### Assessment of vision in people with dementia

There are some simple screening tests that can be used to detect visual dysfunction in patients with dementia (Mancil, 1994):
- ask the patient to read a paragraph from a newspaper or magazine
- ask the patient to copy a line drawing
- show the patient a picture and ask them to describe what they see
- ask the patient to identify photographs of famous people
- ask the patient to reach for objects held up in front and to the side of them
- ask the patient to look at and name colors.

In order to test specific areas of visual loss or dysfunction, contrast sensitivity should be tested, as well as visual acuity and visual fields, and the optic disc should be visualized.

## Interventions for visual dysfunction in dementia

Interventions to improve vision include correction of refractive errors and cataract surgery. These have been recommended as prophylactic or adjunctive treatments for visual hallucinations in patients with probable AD (Chapman et al., 1999). However, it should be noted that caution is needed with vision correction, as a recent study indicates that in frail older people comprehensive vision and eye assessment with appropriate treatment does not always reduce, and may even increase, the risk of falls and fractures (Cumming et al., 2007). A recent study by Cronin-Golomb and associates suggests that enhancement of stimulus strength, such as improved lighting, can ameliorate vision-based deficits and lead to an improvement in some aspects of cognitive performance (Cronin-Golomb et al., 2007).

## Recommendations

1. Be aware that visual dysfunction may be a presenting symptom of dementia, particularly AD. Older adults with persistent visual complaints not attributable to structural eye problems may benefit from referral to a neurologist or geriatrician.
2. Be aware that during the course of dementia, visual problems may arise that can have a significant impact on the performance of assessment tasks, and on function in ADL. Ask the patient with dementia about visual symptoms.
3. A review by optometrist or ophthalmologist should be undertaken early in the disease process, to address refractive errors, check intraocular pressures, and assess for the presence of cataracts.
4. Visual acuity and contrast sensitivity may be improved by the correction of conditions such as cataracts, and making environmental changes such as improved lighting and the use of high-contrast markers.
5. People with the later stages of dementia should be encouraged to continue using their spectacles, which should be clearly labelled for identification.

---

### Case studies

Mr. G is a 74-year-old man who was seen in the memory clinic after presenting with short-term memory problems and difficulty using his computer. He had always been computer literate but was becoming unable to manipulate the mouse and had also experienced problems reading text. He no longer drove a car, and said that he had made the decision to stop driving 18 months earlier when cars coming toward him often seemed to be very distorted in shape. At that time he had been referred to an optometrist, who was unable to find anything to explain his visual problems. He said that since that time he felt he could not always trust his eyesight, as he would feel that the ground was dropping away from him when he was walking, and steps and stairs appeared distorted. He had not had any falls but was worried that he might so he restricted his walking outside to when he was accompanied. On cognitive testing he had clear deficits in short-term memory and difficulties with any cognitive tasks involving visuo-spatial skills. Mr. G was diagnosed with early AD.

Mr. H is a 67-year-old man with early AD who was participating in a clinical drug trial for dementia. On physical examination and visual field testing at the begin-ning of the trial he was found to have a left upper quadrantanopia (not seeing any object that was in his left upper field of vision) but was not aware of this. Magnetic resonance imaging showed no abnormalities. Mr. H was followed up after 3 months by an ophthalmologist and the quadrantanopia remained consist-ent on confrontation assessment of visual fields. Repeat neuroimaging showed no abnormalities, and Mr. H remained free of any visual symptoms.

## Key points

- Symptoms of visual dysfunction may occur before cognitive symptoms in Alzheimer's disease and other dementias.
- Symptoms include blurred and distorted vision, difficulty recognizing familiar objects or faces, difficulty locating familiar objects, difficulty reading or writ-ing, and hallucinations.
- Symptoms may be due to changes in visual acuity and contrast sensitivity, deficits in visuospatial function and color vision, and visual field defects.
- Visual dysfunction is likely to be due to dementia-associated changes in the cerebral cortex, and the retina and optic nerve.

## References

Armstrong, R.A. (1996). Visual field defects in Alzheimer's disease patients may reflect differential pathology in the primary visual cortex. *Optometry & Vision Science*, 73, 677–682.

Baker, D.R., Mendez, M.F., Townsend, J.C., Ilsen, P.F., Bright, D.C. (1997). Optometric management of patients with Alzheimer's disease. *Journal of the American Optometric Association*, 68, 483–494.

Bassi, C.J., Solomon, K., Young, D. (1993). Vision in aging and dementia. *Optometry & Vision Science*, 70, 809–813.

Benson, D.F., Davis, R.J., Snyder, B.D. (1988). Posterior cortical atrophy. *Archives of Neurology*, 45, 789–793.

Berisha, R., Feke G.T., Trempe, C.L, McMeel, J.W., Schepens, C.L. (2007). Retinal abnormalities in early Alzheimer's disease. *Investigative Ophthalmology & Visual Science*, 48, 2285–2289.

Blanks, J.C., Torigoe, Y., Hinton, D.R., Blanks, R.H.I. (1991). Retinal degeneration in the macula of patients with Alzheimer's disease. *Annals of the New York Academy of Sciences*, 640, 44–46.

Boxer, A.L., Kramer, J.H., Du, A.T. et al. (2003). Focal right inferotemporal atrophy in dementia with disproportionate visual constructive impairment. *Neurology*, 61, 1485–1491.

Brazis, P.W., Lee, A.G., Graff-Radford, N., Desai, N.P., Eggenberger, E.R. (2000). Homonymous visual field defects in patients without corresponding structural lesions on neuroimaging. *Journal of Neuro-Ophthalmology*, 20, 92–96.

Butter, C.M., Trobe, J.D., Foster, N.L. (1996). Visual-spatial deficits expalin visual symptoms in Alzheimer's disease. *American Journal of Ophthalmology*, 122, 97–105.

Chapman, F.M., Dickinson, J., McKeith, I., Ballard, C. (1999). Association among visual hallucinations, visual acuity, and specific eye pathologies in Alzheimer's disease: treatment implications. *American Journal of Psychiatry*, 156, 1983–1985.

Collerton, D., Burn, D., McKeith, I., O'Brien, J. (2003). Systematic review and meta-analysis show that dementia with Lewy bodies is a visual-perceptual and attentional-executive dementia. [Erratum appears in *Dement Geriatr Cogn Disord.* (2005). 19, 56]. *Dementia & Geriatric Cognitive Disorders*, 16, 229–237.

Cooper, S.A., Murray, K.L., Heath, C.A., Will, R.G., Knight, R.S.G. (2005). Isolated visual symptoms at onset in spordementiaic Creutzfeldt-Jakob disease: the clinical phenotype of the Heidenhain variant. *British Journal of Ophthalmology*, 89, 1341–1342.

Cormack, F.K., Tovee, M., Ballard, C. (2000). Contrast sensitivity and visual acuity in patients with Alzheimer's disease. *International Journal of Geriatric Psychiatry*, 15, 614–620.

Cronin-Golomb, A. (1995). Vision in Alzheimer's disease. *Gerontologist*, 35, 370–376.

Cronin-Golomb, A., Corkin, S., Growdon, J. (1995). Visual dysfunction predicts cognitive deficits in Alzheimer's disease. *Optometry & Vision Science*, 72, 168–176.

Cronin-Golomb, A., Corkin, S., Rizzo, J.F., Cohen, J., Growdon, J.H., Banks, K.S. (1991). Visual dysfunction in Alzheimer's disease: relation to normal aging. [Erratum appears in *Annals of Neurology*, (1991) 29, 271]. *Annals of Neurology*, 29, 41–52.

Cronin-Golomb, A., Gilmore, G.C., Neargarder, S., Morrison, S., Laudate, T. (2007). Enhanced stimulus strength improves visual cognition in aging and Alzheimer's disease. *Cortex*, 43, 952–966.

Cumming, R.G., Ivers, R., Clemson, L., et al. (2007). Improving vision to prevent falls in frail older people: a randomized trial. *Journal of the American Geriatrics Society*, 55, 175–181.

Cumurciuc, R., Massin, P., Paques, M., et al. (2004). Retinal abnormalities in CADASIL: a retrospective study of 18 patients. *Journal of Neurology, Neurosurgery & Psychiatry*, 75, 1058–1060.

Danesh-Meyer, H.V., Birch, H., Ku, J.Y.F., Carroll, S., Gamble, G. (2006). Reduction of optic nerve fibers in patients with Alzheimer disease identified by laser imaging. *Neurology*, 67, 1852–1854.

de Seze, J., Hache, J.C., Vermeche, P., et al. (1998). Creutzfeldt-Jakob disease: neurophysiologic visual impairments. *Neurology*, 51, 962–967.

Devos, D., Tir, M., Maurage, C.A., et al. (2005). ERG and anatomical abnormalities suggesting retinopathy in dementia with Lewy bodies. *Neurology*, 65, 1107–1110.

Fernandez, R., Kavcic, V., Duffy, C.J. (2007). Neurophysiologic analyses of low- and high-level visual processing in Alzheimer disease. *Neurology*, 68, 2066–2076.

Fujimori, M., Imamura, T., Yamashita, H., Hirono, N., Mori, E. (1997). The disturbances of object vision and spatial vision in Alzheimer's disease. *Dementia & Geriatric Cognitive Disorders*, 8, 228–231.

Geldmacher, D. (2003). Visuospatial dysfunction in the neurogenerative diseases. *Frontiers in BioScience*, 8, e428–e436.

Giannakopoulos, P., Gold, G., Duc, M., Michel, J.P., Hof, P.R., Bouras, C. (1999). Neuroanatomic correlates of visual agnosia in Alzheimer's disease: a clinicopathologic study. *Neurology*, 52, 71–77.

Gilmore, G.C. and Levy J.A. (1991). Spatial contrast sensitivity in Alzheimer's disease: a comparison of two methods. *Optometry & Vision Science*, 68, 790–794.

Gilmore, G.C. and Whitehouse P.J. (1995). Contrast sensitivity in Alzheimer's disease: a 1-year longitudinal analysis. *Optometry & Vision Science*, 72, 83–91.

Goldstein, L.E., Muffat, J.A., Cherney, R.A., et al. (2003). Cytosolic beta-amyloid deposition and supranuclear cataracts in lenses from people with Alzheimer's disease. *Lancet*, 361, 1258–1265.

Gussekloo, J., de Craen, A.J., Oduber, C., van Boxtel, M.P., Westendorp, R.G. (2005). Sensory impairment and cognitive functioning in oldest-old subjects: the Leiden 85+ Study. *American Journal of Geriatric Psychiatry*, 13, 781–786.

Hinton, D. R., Sadun, A.A., Blanks, J.C., Miller, A.C. (1986). Optic-nerve degeneration in Alzheimer's disease. *New England Journal of Medicine*, 315, 485–487.

Hof, P.R., Vogt, B.A., Bouras, C., Morrison, J.A. (1997). Atypical form of Alzheimer's disease with prominent posterior cortical atrophy: a review of lesion distribution and circuit disconnection in cortical visual pathways. *Vision Research*, 37, 3609–3625.

Holroyd, S.M.D. and Sheldon-Keller A.P.D. (1995). A study of visual hallucinations in Alzheimer's Disease. *American Journal of Geriatric Psychiatry*, 3, 198–205.

Hutton, J.T., Morris, J.L., Elias, J.W., Poston, J.N. (1993). Contrast sensitivity dysfunction in Alzheimer's disease. *Neurology*, 43, 2328–2330.

Iseri, P.K., Altinas, O., Tokay, T., Yuksel, N. (2006). Relationship between cognitive impairment and retinal morphological and visual functional abnormalities in Alzheimer disease. *Journal of Neuro-Ophthalmology*, 26, 18–24.

Kaskie, B. and Storandt, M. (1995). Visuospatial deficit in dementia of the Alzheimer type. *Archives of Neurology*, 52, 422–425.

Katz, B. and S. Rimmer. (1989). Ophthalmologic manifestations of Alzheimer's disease. *Survey of Ophthalmology*, 34, 31–43.

Keri, S., Antal, A., Kalman, J., Janka, Z., Benedek, G. (1999). Early visual impairment is independent of the visuocognitive and memory disturbances in Alzheimer's disease. *Vision Research*, 39, 2261–2265.

Koch, J.M., Datta, G., Makhdoom, S., Grossberg, G.T. (2005). Unmet visual needs of Alzheimer's disease patients in long-term care facilities. *Journal of the. American Medical Directors Association*, 6, 233–237.

Koronyo-Hamaoui, M. Koronyo, Y., Ljubimov, A., et al. (2011). Identification of amyloid plaques in retinas from Alzheimer's patients and noninvasive *in vivo* optical imaging of retinal plaques in a mouse model. *NeuroImage*, 54, S204–S217.

Kropp, S., Schulz-Schaeffer, W.J., Finkenstaedt, M., et al. (1999). The Heidenhain variant of Creutzfeldt-Jakob disease. *Archives of Neurology*, 56, 55–61.

Lakshminarayanan, V., Lagrave, J., Kean, M.L., Dick, M., Shankle, R. (1996). Vision in dementia: contrast effects. *Neurological Research*, 18, 9–15.

Lee, A.G. and Martin C.O. (2004). Neuro-ophthalmic findings in the visual variant of Alzheimer's disease. *Ophthalmology*, 111, 376–380; discussion 380–381.

Mancil, G.L. (1994). Visual disorders associated with Alzheimer's disease and optometric management. *Journal of the American Optometric Association*, 65, 27–31.

McShane, R., Gedling, K., Reading, M., McDonald, B., Esiri, M., Hope, T. (1995). Prospective study of relations between cortical Lewy bodies, poor eyesight, and hallucinations in Alzheimer's disease. *Journal of Neurology, Neurosurgery & Psychiatry*, 59, 185–188.

Mendez, M.F., Cherrier, M.M., Cymerman, J.S. (1997). Hemispatial neglect on visual search tasks in Alzheimer's disease. *Neuropsychiatry, Neuropsychology, & Behavioral Neurology*, 10, 203–208.

Mendez, M.F., Ghajarania, M., Perryman, K.M. (2002). Posterior cortical atrophy: clinical characteristics and differences compared to Alzheimer's disease. *Dementia & Geriatric Cognitive Disorders*, 14, 33–40.

Mendez, M.F., Mendez, M.A., Martin, R., Smyth, K.A., Whitehouse, P.J. (1990). Complex visual disturbances in Alzheimer's disease. *Neurology*, 40, 439–443.

Mendola, J.D., Cronin-Golomb, A., Corkin, S., Growdon, J. (1995). Prevalence of visual deficits in Alzheimer's disease. *Optometry & Vision Science*, 72, 155–167.

Mielke, R., Kessler, J., Fink, G., Herholz, K., Heiss, W. (1995). Dysfunction of visual cortex contributes to disturbed processing of visual information in Alzheimer's disease. *International Journal of Neuroscience*, 82, 1–9.

Morrison, J.H., Hof, P.R., Bouras, C. (1991). An anatomic substrate for visual disconnection in Alzheimer's disease. *Annals of the New York Academy of Sciences*, 640, 36–43.

Murgatroyd, C. and Prettyman, R. (2001). An investigation of visual hallucinosis and visual sensory status in dementia. *International Journal of Geriatric Psychiatry*, 16, 709–713.

Nobili, L. and Sannita W.G. (1997). Cholinergic modulation, visual function and Alzheimer's dementia. *Vision Research*, 37, 3559–3571.

Pache, M., Smeets, C.H., Fontana Gasio, P., et al. (2003). Colour vision deficiencies in Alzheimer's disease. *Age & Ageing*, 32, 422–426.

Paquet, C., Boissonnot, M., Roger, F., Dighiero, P., Gil, R., Hugon, J. (2007). Abnormal retinal thickness in patients with mild cognitive impairment and Alzheimer's disease. *Neuroscience Letters*, 420, 97–99.

Pham, T.Q., Kifley, A., Alexander, G.E., et al. (2006). Relation of age-related macular degeneration and cognitive impairment in an older population. *Gerontology*, 52, 353–358.

Pietrini, P., Furey, M.L., et al. (1996). Preferential metabolic involvement of visual cortical areas in a subtype of Alzheimer's disease: clinical implications. *American Journal of Psychiatry*, 153, 1261–1268.

Pliskin, N.H., Kiolbasa, T.A., Towle, V.L., et al. (1996). Charles Bonnet syndrome: an early marker for dementia?. *Journal of the American Geriatrics Society*, 44, 1055–1061.

Ravaglia, S., Costa, A., Santorelli, F.M., Nappi, G., Moglia, A. (2004). Retinal migraine as unusual feature of cerebral autosomal dominant arteriopathy with subcortical infarcts and leukoencephalopathy (CADASIL). *Cephalalgia*, 24, 74–77.

Rizzo, J.F., Cronin-Golomb, A., Growdon, J.H., et al. (1992). Retinocalcarine function in Alzheimer's disease. A clinical and electrophysiological study. *Archives of Neurology*, 49, 93–101.

Rizzo, M., Anderson, S.W., Dawson, J., Nawrot, M. (2000). Vision and cognition in Alzheimer's disease. *Neuropsychologia*, 38, 1157–1169.

Saliba, D., Solomon, D., Rubenstein, L., et al. (2004). Quality indicators for the management of medical conditions in nursing home residents. *Journal of the American Medical Directors Association*, 5, 297–309.

Schmidtke, K., Hull, M., Talazko, J. (2005). Posterior cortical atrophy: variant of Alzheimer's disease? A case series with PET findings. *Journal of Neurology*, 252, 27–35.

Tay, T., Wang, J.J., Kifley, A., Lindley, R., Newall, P., Mitchell, P. (2006). Sensory and cognitive association in older persons: findings from an older Australian population. *Gerontology*, 52, 386–394.

Tetewsky, S.J. and Duffy, C.J. (1999). Visual loss and getting lost in Alzheimer's disease. *Neurology*, 52, 958–965.

Trick, G.L., Trick, L.R., Morris, P., Wolf, M. (1995). Visual field loss in senile dementia of the Alzheimer's type. *Neurology*, 45, 68–74.

Victoroff, J., Ross, G.W., Benson, F., Verity, A., Vinters, H.V. (1994). Posterior cortical atrophy. Neuropathologic correlations. *Archives of Neurology*, 51, 269–274.

# 9

# Oral disease

## Introduction

Recent advances in preventive dentistry and the retention of natural teeth into older age mean that more people will require dental attention as they age. As a large proportion of these older people will have dementia, it is important that there be an integration of oral hygiene and dental care into health-care planning for people with dementia.

Worldwide studies report an increased incidence of poor oral hygiene and increased tooth caries in the dementia population compared with those individuals without dementia, in both community dwellings and residential care (Chalmers et al., 2005, Chen et al., 2010). In addition to generally poor oral hygiene, dementia patients have been found to have a decreased number of natural teeth (Miura et al., 2003), with the incidence of denture use lower in edentulous individuals with dementia than in those without dementia (Syrjala et al., 2006). Dementia patients are also seen with higher levels of plaque and calculus load compared with older people with no dementia, and the prevalence of xerostomia (dry mouth) has also been reported to be higher in the dementia population, due to a combination of physiological changes in saliva production and medication use (Ship and Puckett, 1994).

The benefits of good oral health should be emphasized for its positive effects on general health, self-esteem and dignity, and nutrition. It is also important for social interaction, as the negative effects of missing or decaying teeth, gingivitis, and halitosis are significant. Undiagnosed and untreated dental disease can significantly affect an individual's quality of life and behavior. Poor oral health greatly impacts on an individual's general health, with the potential development of a number of conditions including poor nutrition, dehydration, oral and systemic infections, and aspiration pneumonia, which may all in turn impact negatively on cognition (Goodman et al., 1993).

## Epidemiology of oral disease in dementia

Older people in residential aged care facilities appear to be particularly at risk of oral disease. A study estimating oral health status and dental treatment needs in 348 nursing-home residents in Western Australia (half of whom had dementia) found that the vast majority of residents had poor oral health, with a high need for dental treatment (Stubbs and Riordan, 2002). The inadequacy of oral hygiene was noted by Montal and colleagues (2006) in an observational study of 320 nursing-home patients in southern France. They found that only 40% of residents had satisfactory oral hygiene. Similar findings were noted by Wyatt and colleagues (2006) in a study of Canadian nursing-home residents.

Chalmers and colleagues (2002b) examined 224 residents in nursing homes in South Australia in a cross-sectional study of the prevalence of oral disease. They found that 66% of the residents were edentulous, and that there was a corresponding very high level of dental caries and plaque accumulation in those dentate residents with a diagnosis of dementia. In a second longitudinal study, they assessed the dental health of 232 community-dwelling older people both with and without dementia, and showed that there was a significantly higher incidence of coronal and root caries in those with dementia than in those without dementia (Chalmers et al., 2002a). The characteristics associated with a high level of caries included the person being in the later stages of dementia, being of male gender, experiencing oral hygiene difficulties, the carer experiencing a high level of burden, and the use of neuroleptic medication.

Recently a study by Ellefsen et al. (2008) examined the prevalence of dental caries in 106 community-dwelling patients, of whom 87 had dementia. Patients with a diagnosis of Alzheimer's disease (AD) had a significantly higher number of caries than patients with other dementia diagnoses or those without dementia. It appeared that even before the diagnosis of dementia was made, active dental caries were present. However, at the 1-year follow-up of these patients, those with a dementia diagnosis other than AD had a higher risk of developing multiple caries during the year after the diagnosis was made (Ellefsen et al., 2009).

## The impact of dementia on oral health

The negative effects of dementia on oral health have been known for many years. An early observational study in 1987 of residents in a number of nursing facilities in Los Angeles found a higher number of older people with dementia had very poor oral hygiene and chronic periodontal disease compared with older people without dementia (Friedlander and Jarvik, 1987). Problems with inserting partial dental prostheses were noted, as were the high numbers of lost or damaged dentures and prostheses. The anticholinergic effects of antipsychotic medication were also discussed, with xerostomia considered a major problem. The benchmark study by Ship (1992) also found poor oral hygiene in people with AD compared with community controls without dementia. In particular, Ship found a significant correlation between increased periodontal pocketing and decreasing cognition. Jones and colleagues (1993) reported similar findings in a study of male veterans with and without dementia. In this study, subjects with dementia were noted to have significantly higher numbers of surfaces with decay at baseline compared with subjects without dementia, with a doubling of the incidence of caries over a 1-year follow-up period.

There is an interesting link between having a low number of teeth and the development of dementia, with Stein et al. (2007) showing a strong association between these two factors. Stein found a connection between a low number of remaining teeth and the subsequent risk of developing dementia in 144 participants in a longitudinal study of aging and dementia (the Nun Study). In ten years of follow-up, those participants with the fewest teeth had the highest risk of developing dementia. Inflammation has been suggested as playing a role in the pathophysiology of AD, and the high levels of inflammatory markers such as interleukin-1 and interleukin-6 seen in periodontal disease may contribute to this. Stewart and Hirani (2007) showed the same strong association between poor dentition and cognitive impairment in their analysis of data from the Health Survey for England 2000. However, the association was only significant among community-dwelling older people, and not in those residents of care homes. Although a relationship has been established between dementia and poor oral health, it remains unclear as to whether the link is casual or causal.

The effects on oral health of the increasing cognitive impairment and decreasing function that occur in dementia are multifactorial. With a disturbance in executive functioning comes impaired planning and organization, and a loss of motivation ensues. The ability to initiate tasks then decreases as the disease progresses, resulting in an increased reliance on carers, thus also increasing the risk of oral disease (Ghezzi and Ship, 2000). There is deterioration in the patient's ability to self-care, along with an impaired ability to learn new information, or to adapt to changes such as dental prostheses. The difficulty in following instructions means that prompting may not be adequate for promoting oral hygiene, so full assistance may be necessary (Syrjala et al., 2006). Apraxia and agnosia result in a worsening of voluntary motor skills, such as using a toothbrush or squeezing toothpaste out of a tube, and there is an inability to recognize familiar items or to remember how to use them correctly (Chiapelli et al., 2006). A decrease in both expressive and receptive communication skills results in difficulty in reporting dental discomfort or pain, and in understanding the need for assistance with oral care (Kocaelli et al., 2002).

Changes in behavior also impact upon oral health. There may be an increase in combative behaviors such as aggression and agitation, with subsequent resistance to personal care, including oral care (Friedlander et al., 2006). Alternatively, apathy may also lead to resistance to care, or the requirement for full assistance with care. If there is an increased carer burden, then carer stress increases, with an associated decrease in motivation to overcome the patient's resistance to care (Chalmers et al., 2002a). A decrease in oral fluid intake and subsequent dehydration can also lead to xerostomia and an increase in dental disease (Ship, 1992).

Although xerostomia is a very common problem, sialorrhea (drooling) may also be a problem in the later stages of the disease. This is likely to be related to dysphagia, and to sitting with the head tilted forwards, and may be exacerbated by discomfort or pain due to oral disease (Fiske, 2006). Another problem that may occur later in the disease is the emergence of sucking reflexes, and involuntary oral movements including overactive tongue movements, making the delivery of oral care very difficult (Nordenram et al., 1997).

Having dementia is itself a factor that decreases oral health maintenance, as shown by Vehkalahti and colleagues (1996), who found the presence of dementia was a highly significant factor in dental consultation nonparticipation. A study of carers of people with dementia found that the carers were worried about taking people with dementia to the dentist because of possible behavioral problems (Hilton and Simons, 2003).

## The impact of medication on oral health in dementia

Medications used by people with dementia can significantly influence their oral health, and it is important that dentists are aware of the drugs their patients are taking (Carter et al., 2007). Prescription drugs may have specific side effects such as xerostomia, stomatitis, or tardive dyskinesia, or specific adverse effects such as osteonecrosis of the jaw, which may occur following dental extractions. In their study of 85 community-dwelling people with dementia, Chapman and Shaw (1991) found an increased risk of developing tooth caries and periodontal disease in individuals taking common prescription medication, compared with those people with dementia taking no medication (Chapman and Shaw, 1991).

Antipsychotic and anticonvulsant medications together with other anticholinergic medications have been linked to the dysfunction of the salivary glands, leading to xerostomia. Other medications that can also potentially cause xerostomia include diuretics such as furosemide, lithium, ACE inhibitors, antihistamines, antidepressants such as citalopram, and tricyclic antidepressants such as amitriptyline. Studies of otherwise healthy dementia patients taking no medication have also found a decrease in saliva production, suggesting that those people with dementia may already be compromized in terms of reduced salivary gland function (Goodman et al., 1993). Without the antibacterial, lubricating, remineralizing, and buffering effects of saliva, the risk of plaque accumulation increases, resulting in problems with dentures, and an increased likelihood of tooth caries and periodontal disease, the results of which can then compromise the nutritional intake of dementia patients (Chalmers et al., 2005, Fiske, 2006).

Other medication-related problems include gingival hyperplasia and possibly oral ulceration that can occur with anticonvulsants such as phenytoin, and special care is needed when prescribing anticonvulsant medication, particularly where poor oral hygiene exists (Niessen and Jones, 1987). Syrup-based medications that are high in sugar may increase the risk of dental caries, whereas the cholinesterase inhibitors may cause glossitis (Ettinger, 2000), and oral candidiasis may occur with antibiotics, particularly in the presence of poor oral hygiene.

## Symptoms and signs of oral disease in dementia

Patients in the early stages of dementia are usually able to describe their symptoms and express their needs. However, as the disease progresses, this can become difficult and patients may be unable to interpret their own discomfort or pain. For these patients it is important that the family or professional carer is able to recognize changes in behavior, or recognize other signs that may indicate the presence of dental problems (Fiske, 2006).

Common symptoms and signs of oral disease may include:
- refusing to eat or drink
- refusing to open their mouth
- moaning or shouting
- restlessness and agitation
- halitosis
- holding or pulling at their face
- drooling and spitting
- bleeding from the gums, tongue, or cheeks
- refusing to wear previously worn full or partial dentures
- disturbed sleep
- refusing to allow toothbrushing or mouthwashes
- aggressive behavior.

The appearance of any of these symptoms or signs should alert carers to the possibility of active oral disease.

## Management of oral disease in dementia

The literature strongly supports the integration of oral health care into the multidisciplinary approach to dementia care. Geriatricians should ideally include an evaluation of oral health status as part of a comprehensive geriatric assessment (Weyant et al., 2004). Several studies suggest that assessment and care planning should begin at the time dementia is diagnosed, before the disease progresses and the patient becomes less able to cooperate (Kocaelli et al., 2002, Adam and Preston, 2006, Chiappelli et al., 2006, Fiske, 2006, Ellefsen et al., 2008). These studies acknowledge the difficulty in treating patients as their ability to cooperate and tolerate treatment diminishes with their decline in cognition.

## Goals of oral health care

There are a number of recommended outcomes that should be achieved with good oral health care in people with dementia (Jones et al., 2000). These include freedom from oral pain, having a safe oral environment with a low risk of aspiration, having emergency dental care available if needed, preventing mouth infections, having daily mouth care as much a part of personal care as brushing the hair, preventing discomfort from loose teeth or sore gums, brushing teeth daily, having staff provide oral hygiene as needed, and recognizing oral problems early. Being able to taste food, chew and enjoy eating, being able to speak normally, having a normal facial appearance, and having fresh breath to allow social behavior such as kissing to occur have also been included as goals of treatment (Nordenram et al., 1994). A longitudinal study in a geriatric dental clinic has shown that with appropriate dental treatment, people with dementia were able to maintain their dentition and oral function with similar patterns of tooth loss to people without dementia (Chen et al., 2010).

## Assessment and treatment

The oral health assessment of a person with dementia should not only include examination of the mouth and teeth, but should also consider previous dental history, preventive behavior, current oral hygiene practices, and medical history and current medications. The stage of dementia and any concomitant behavior that might make the implementation of oral care difficult should also be noted (Fiske, 2006).

The extent of involvement of the carer in the provision of oral health needs to be documented, as the carer is likely to be the main provider of oral health care – therefore their knowledge and understanding of oral hygiene and their ability or inability to provide care will impact greatly on the person with dementia (Hugo et al., 2007). Training of the family carer in good oral hygiene techniques is important (Ghezzi and Ship, 2000). Also important, however, is ensuring the carer can find a balance between encouraging independence in self-performance of oral hygiene and providing that care in order to ensure that it occurs.

Patients with early dementia should have a full assessment from their own dentist, as cooperation with treatment is not usually a problem at this stage of the disease. The development of a flexible and individualized oral health-care plan early in the disease process that focuses on prevention and retention of natural teeth is likely to reduce patient stress and the need for emergency treatment later in the disease (Fiske, 2006).

It is important that the dentist is aware of the diagnosis of dementia so that treatment can be planned accordingly. The goals for dental treatment in people with dementia will depend on the stage of the patient's dementia. In the early stages of dementia treatment should focus on active management of any oral disease and restoration of good oral health. As dementia progresses, the treatment focus should shift toward maintenance of oral health and dentition and the prevention of disease (Niessen and Jones, 1987). Daily care of the teeth should include twice-daily brushing with a fluoridated toothpaste. Macentee (2000) suggests the use of a chlorhexidine mouthwash to control caries, and notes that chlorhexidine gel, together with fluoride gel has been shown to reduce the incidence of caries in younger adults at risk of oral disease.

In the later stages of dementia, the patient may not be able to describe symptoms of oral disease, so it is important that conditions such as gingivitis, mouth ulceration, glossitis, oral candidiasis, and angular stomatitis be recognized and treated to relieve mouth discomfort.

Chalmers (2006) has written extensively on the subject of minimal intervention dentistry for older patients, with the focus of treatment on early detection and prevention of oral disease, aiming to preserve as much of the natural tooth structure as possible through promotion of external and internal remineralization, and surgical intervention only after disease has been controlled. She describes the various techniques and materials available to dentists to manage older people with significant oral disease.

For patients with dementia who are admitted to a residential-care facility, it is recommended that the patient's general practitioner perform an oral health assessment on admission. If this cannot occur, nursing staff trained in oral-health assessment should complete the assessment. Dental-hygiene education for nursing staff in residential-care facilities has been shown to be effective in improving dental hygiene among residents (Kullberg et al., 2010). In Australia, the Federal Government has developed evidence-based oral health planning guidelines for people in residential care. These include education and learning materials to enable staff to carry out assessments using the Oral Health Assessment Tool for Dental Screening, to recognize oral disease, and to know when referral to a dentist is required (*Better Oral Health in Residential Care*, 2009 (South Australian Dental Service, 2009). There is detailed information on the provision of oral hygiene for residents with their own teeth and for those with dentures. The guidelines also include information on managing difficult behavior, and consent issues.

When a person with dementia requires a dental consultation, it is recommended that the same dentist is always visited for consistency. It is important that the appointments are kept short, that they occur at the time of the day when the person with dementia is most alert and cooperative (usually in the morning), and that a carer attends to provide a familiar voice and reassurance, and to understand what treatment is occurring (Chiapelli et al., 2006).

Sedation has been recommended as a management tool for patients with advanced dementia when oral treatment is required, as this alleviates difficulties in managing resitant behavior. Although removing decayed teeth is generally seen as preferable to complex restorative procedures (Adam and Preston, 2006), Nordenram and colleagues (1997) have instead suggested that the preservation of natural teeth may maintain a better quality of life, even if there is minimal impact on nutrition. It is suggested that this occurs because mechanoreceptive nerve terminals located in the periodontal ligaments of teeth transmit spatial information and details of tooth load, which may be linked to a form of chewing memory that helps dementia patients retain the ability to chew longer into the onset of disease progression.

## Recommendations

1. Patients with cognitive impairment or early dementia should be referred for a dental consultation and review with the aim of maintaining good oral health, or restoring good oral health.
2. A regime of twice-daily teeth and gum brushing should be instituted. A soft toothbrush with high fluoride toothpaste is recommended. Spitting rather than rinsing the mouth after brushing allows optimal action of the fluoride.
3. Dentures should be cleaned twice daily (out of the mouth) to remove plaque. The gums should be gently cleaned with a soft brush, and dentures should stay soaking in cold water overnight. Dentures should be disinfected weekly.
4. Avoid the complications of a dry mouth by encouraging regular sips or drinks of water, and the use of saliva stimulators such as lemon-flavored tooth-friendly sweets, or saliva substitutes such as mouth gel or spray.
5. If patients resist oral hygiene measures, consider using a mouthwash or gel containing chlorhexidine to help reduce caries.
6. Consider the effect of medication on oral health, particularly antipsychotics, anticonvulsants, and anticholinergic medications.
7. Consider use of adequate sedation for dental work, particularly in the later stages of dementia.
8. Provide education to family and professional carers on an appropriate oral hygiene routine for the person for whom they care. Care should be tailored to the patient's stage of dementia.

---

### Case studies

Mr. D is a 55-year-old man who attended the memory clinic for review of his memory problems. Mr. D, who lives with his wife, reported problems at work due to his memory loss, and his family had also noticed he was forgetting appointments and repeating himself. After a diagnosis of AD was confirmed, he was commenced on a cholinesterase inhibitor and 6-monthly follow-up was recommended. At the next visit Mrs. D expressed concerns about her husband's refusal to wear his partial denture, and its effect on his appearance and nutrition. Mr. D gave vague reasons to explain this change in behavior, saying "I am not going out, so no one will see me," "it's not clean," and finally "it does not fit any more." On examination, Mr. D had three broken lower molars and significant plaque build-up. Referral to the family dentist was recommended. Reconstruction and cleaning was completed over four visits, resulting in Mr. D resuming the wearing of his partial denture. Mrs. D remained vigilant and provided reminders to her husband to clean his teeth and use mouthwash daily. Acting early in the disease process has allowed Mr. D to consent to treatment and fully cooperate with the treating dentist.

Mr. L is an 83-year-old man who lives alone in his own home. He has moderate dementia and receives support from community services for housekeeping, including cooking and shopping. He had declined any input from community nursing services or medical practitioners, and was noted by one of the care workers to have foul-smelling breath and to be drooling. He was only eating soft food. He developed a fever and gastroenteritis and was brought to hospital by a care worker. He was found to have severe gingivitis and a dental abscess. After intravenous antibiotic therapy he required extensive dental intervention under general anaesthetic in an attempt to preserve as many teeth as possible. Although several extractions were required, the dentist was able to keep the majority of Mr. L's natural teeth, allowing him to be able to eat most kinds of food. Following discharge from hospital, the care workers visiting him were taught how to assist him to clean his teeth at least once daily.

## Key points

- Poor oral health is more common in people with dementia than in people without dementia.
- Changes may occur before the diagnosis of dementia is made.
- Oral disease occurring in dementia includes increased plaque accumulation and caries, fewer retained natural teeth, dry mouth, and less use of dentures.
- Oral disease in dementia is due to many factors, including poor self-care, inability to follow instructions, decreased executive function, increasing dyspraxia and agnosia, and behavioral problems.

## References

Adam, H. and Preston, A. (2006). The oral health of individuals with dementia in nursing homes, *Gerodontology*, 23, 99–105.

Carter, L., McHenry, I., Godlington, F., Meechan, J. (2007). Prescribed medication taken by patients attending general dental practice: changes over 20 years. *British Dental Journal*, 203, E8. DOI: 10.1038/bdj.2007.629.

Chalmers, J. (2006). Minimal intervention dentistry: Part 1. Strategies for addressing the new caries challenge in older patients. *Journal of the Canadian Dental Association*, 72, 427–433.

Chalmers, J.M., Carter, K.D., Spencer, A.J. (2002a). Caries incidence and increments in community-living older adults with and without dementia. *Gerodontology*, 19, 80–94.

Chalmers, J., Hodge, C., Fuss, J., Spencer, A., Carter, K. (2002b). The prevalence and experience of oral diseases in Adelaide nursing home residents. *Australian Dental Journal*, 47, 123–130.

Chalmers, J.M., Carter, K.D., Spencer, A.J. (2005). Caries incidence and increments in Adelaide nursing homes residents. *Gerodontology*, 19, 30–40.

Chapman, P.J. and Shaw, R.M. (1991). Normative dental treatment needs of Alzheimer's patients. *Australian Dental Journal*, 36, 141–144.

Chen X., Shuman S.K., Hodges J.S., et al. (2010). Patterns of tooth loss in older adults with and without dementia: a retrospective study based on a Minnesota cohort. *Journal of the American Geriatrics Society*, 58, 2300–2307.

Chiappelli, F., Manfrini, E., Edgerton, M., et al. (2006). Clinical evidence and evidence-based dental treatment of special populations: patients with Alzheimer's disease. *Journal of the California Dental Association*, 34, 439–447.

Ellefsen, B., Holm-Pederson, P., Morse, D., et al. (2008). Caries prevalence in older persons with and without dementia. *Journal of the American Geriatrics Society*, 56, 59–67.

Ellefsen, B., Holm-Pederson, P., Morse, D., et al. (2009). Assessing caries increments in elderly patients with and without dementia: a one-year follow-up study. *Journal of the American Dental Association*, 140, 1392–1400.

Ettinger, R. (2000). Dental management of patients with Alzheimer's disease and other dementias. *Gerodontology*, 17, 8–16.

Fiske, J. (2006) Guidelines for the development of local standards of oral health care for people with dementia. *Gerodontology*, 23, 5–32.

Friedlander, A. and Jarvik, L. (1987). Dental management of the patient with dementia. *Oral Surgery, Oral Medicine, Oral Pathology*, 64, 549–553.

Friedlander, A., Norman, D., Mahler, M., et al. (2006). Alzheimer's disease: psychopathology, medical management and dental implications. *Journal of the American Dental Association*, 137, 1240–1251.

Ghezzi, E. and Ship, J.A. (2000). Dementia and oral health. *Oral Surgery, Oral Medicine, Oral Pathology, Oral Radiology & Endodontics*, 89, 2–5.

Goodman, H.S., Ickrath, M., Niessen, L. (1993). Managing patients with AD: The primary care role of dentists. *Journal of the American Dental Association*, 124, 75–80.

Hilton, C., and Simons, B. (2003). Dental surgery attendance amongst patients with moderately advanced dementia attending a day unit: a survey of carers' views. *British Dental Journal*, 195, 39–40.

Hugo, F., Hilgert, J., Bertuzzi, D., Padilha, D., De Marchi, R. (2007). Oral health behaviour and socio-demographic profile of subjects with Alzheimer's disease as reported by their family caregivers. *Gerodontology*, 24, 36–40.

Jones, J., Brown, E., Volicer, L. (2000). Target outcomes for long-term oral health care in dementia: a Delphi approach. *Journal of Public Health Dentistry*, 60, 330–334.

Jones, J.A., Lavallee, N., Alman, J., et al. (1993). Caries incidence in patients with dementia. *Gerodontology*, 10, 76–82.

Kocaelli, H., Yaltirik, M., Ilhan, L., et al. (2002) Alzheimer's disease and dental management. *Oral Surgery, Oral Medicine, Oral Pathology, Oral Radiology & Endodontics*, 93, 521–524.

Kullberg, E., Sjogren, P., Forsell, M., et al. (2010). Dental hygiene education for nursing staff in a nursing home for older people. *Journal of Advanced Nursing*, 66, 1273–1279.

MacEntee, M. (2000). Oral care for successful aging in long-term care. *Journal of Public Health Dentistry*, 60, 326–329.

Miura, H., Yamasaki, K., Kariyasu, M., Miura, K., Sumi, Y. (2003). Relationship between cognitive function and mastication in elderly females. *Journal of Oral Rehabilitation*, 30, 808–811.

Montal, S., Tramini, P., Triay, J., et al. (2006). Oral hygiene and the need for treatment of the dependent institutionalised elderly. *Gerodontology*, 23, 67–72.

Niessen, L. and Jones, J. (1987). Professional dental care for patients with dementia. *Gerodontology*, 6, 67–71.

Nordenram, G., Ronngerg, L., Winblad, B. (1994). The perceived importance of appearance and oral function, comfort and health for severely demented persons rated by relatives, nursing staff and hospital dentists. *Gerodontology*, 11, 18–24.

Nordenram, G., Ryd-Kejellen, E., Ericsson, K., et al. (1997). Alzheimer's disease, oral function and nutritional status, *Gerodontology*, 13, 9–16.

Ship, J.A. (1992) Oral health of patients with Alzheimer's disease. *Journal of the American Dental Association*, 123, 53–58.

Ship, J.A. and Puckett, S.A. (1994). Longitudinal study on oral health in subjects with Alzheimer's disease. *Journal of the American Geriatrics Society*, 42, 57–63.

South Australian Dental Service (2009). Better Oral Health in Residential Care. Australian Government Department of Health and Ageing. Adelaide: 2009. Available at: http://www.health.gov.au/internet/main/publishing.nsf/Content/ageing-better-oral-health.htm [Accessed March 2, 2012].

Stein, P., Desrosiers, M., Donegan, S., et al. (2007). Tooth loss, dementia and neuropathology in the Nun Study. *Journal of the American Dental Association*, 138, 1314–1322.

Stewart, R. and Hirani, V. (2007). Dental health and cognitive impairment in an English national survey population. *Journal of the American Geriatrics Society*, 55, 1410–1414.

Stubbs, C., and Riordan, P. (2002). Dental screening of older adults living in residential aged care facilities in Perth. *Australian Dental Journal*, 47, 321–326.

Syrjala, A., Ylostalo, P., Sulkava, R., et al. (2006). Relationship between cognitive impairment and oral health: results of the Health 2000 Health Examination Survey in Finland. *Acta Odontologica Scandinavica*, 65, 103–108.

Vehkalahti, M., Siukosaari, P., Ainamo, A., et al. (1996). Factors related to the non-attendance in a clinical oral health study on the home-dwelling old elderly. *Gerodentology*, 13, 17–24.

Weyant, R.J., Pandav, R.S., Plowman, J.L., et al. (2004). Medical and cognitive cor-relates of denture wearing in older community-dwelling adults. *Journal of the American Geriatrics Society*, 52, 596–600.

Wyatt, C., So, F., Williams, M., et al. (2006). The development, implementation, utilization and outcomes of a comprehensive dental program for older adults residing in long-term care facilities. *Journal of the Canadian Dental Association*, 72, 419–427.

# 10

# Frailty

## Introduction

Frailty is a state of reduced physiological reserves in the domains of physical ability, cognition, and health. This diminishment increases an individual's vulnerability to adverse outcomes, including functional dependence, institutionalization, and death (Rockwood et al., 2000). No single process has been identified to explain frailty, but it is known that frailty increases with age, is more common in women, and is multifactorial in origin, with an interplay of biological, medical, social, and psychological factors (Rockwood et al., 2004). It has been operationalized as a combination of unexplained weight loss, low grip strength, self-reported exhaustion, slow walking speed, and low physical activity (Fried et al., 2001).

Many studies have reported an association between frailty and cognitive impairment, with a higher degree of physical frailty correlating with more severe cognitive impairment. As a consequence it has been suggested that frailty and cognitive impairment may share a common underlying pathogenesis (Buchman et al., 2007). Different studies have demonstrated the relationship between frailty and cognitive impairment in different ways: through cognitive function as a predictor of decline in physical performance (Atkinson et al., 2010); through physical performance measures as predictors of decline in cognitive function (Boyle et al., 2010); and demonstrating concurrent declines in cognitive and physical function (Black and Rush, 2002, Atkinson et al., 2005). The temporal relationship between the onset of frailty, as measured by physical functioning and cognitive decline, remains unclear.

## Epidemiology of frailty in dementia

There is evidence from a number of cohort studies that decreases in muscle strength and walking speed ("frailty") may precede the onset of dementia by many years, and proponents suggest declining motor function as a noncognitive indicator of the progression of subclinical dementia (Alfaro-Acha et al., 2006). A prospective cohort study of 816 older people assessed for both cognitive and motor function found that over 6 years of follow-up, significantly more cases of Alzheimer's disease (AD) developed in those subjects classified as frail at study entry (based on tests of upper and lower limb strength and function), compared with those who were considered non-frail (Aggarwal et al., 2006). They also found that those older people assessed to have mild cognitive impairment (MCI) at study entry had lower levels of motor function compared with those people without cognitive impairment. Lower levels of physical performance were associated with an increased risk of developing dementia in a 6-year prospective cohort study of 2288 older people without dementia at study entry (Wang et al., 2006). Physical performance was scored out of 16 and was assessed by grip strength, standing balance, chair stands, and gait speed. For every 1 point lower on physical performance scored at study entry, there was a 10% associated increase in the risk of developing dementia in the 6-year follow-up period. The authors suggested that higher levels of physical performance might delay the onset of dementia. A 10-year prospective study of 1370 older people with a Mini-Mental State Examination (MMSE) score of 21 or higher at baseline found that those participants assessed as being frail using the criteria of weight loss, slow gait speed, low handgrip strength, self-reported exhaustion, and low physical activity had a significantly greater chance of experiencing cognitive decline in the following 10 years, compared with those who were not found to be frail (Samper-Ternent et al., 2008).

In a prospective longitudinal study, 823 older people without dementia underwent annual assessments of frailty and cognition (Buchman et al., 2007). During 3 years of follow-up, 89 people developed AD, with both the baseline level of frailty and the annual rate of change in degree of frailty associated with an increased risk of developing AD. The same group of study participants was followed for between 6 and 10 years, with the development of MCI in the 761 remaining older people also measured (Boyle et al., 2010). Physical frailty was found to be associated with a higher risk of developing MCI, with greater frailty predicting an increased risk of developing MCI.

A number of studies have found that impaired cognitive function precedes a decline in physical function and development of frailty. Raji and colleagues (2010) found that poor cognition predicted the development of frailty over a 10-year period, and suggested that cognitive decline is a sign of an older person's transition into frailty. They studied a cohort of 942 older people who were not frail at entry into the study, and found that those with poor cognition (with an MMSE score less than 21) at entry had a 9% increased chance each year of becoming frail. Inzitari and colleagues (2007), in a cohort study of 1052 older people, found that those with deficits in attention at study entry showed lower levels of motor performance, including in gait speed and chair stands, at 3-year follow-up.

Several of the core components of frailty, including low gait speed, low muscle strength, and weight loss, have been shown to be individually associated with the development of impaired cognitive function. Waite and colleagues (2005) identified gait slowing as a predictor of dementia in a 6-year prospective cohort study of

630 older people, with those individuals who had both cognitive impairment and gait and motor slowing being 5 times more likely to develop dementia than those without this combination. In a study of 970 older people, Boyle and colleagues (2009) found that a composite measure of muscle strength from 9 muscle groups predicted cognitive decline, with higher strength at baseline associated with a slower rate of decline in cognitive function. In a 7-year prospective study of 2160 older people, Alfaro-Acha and colleagues (2006) found that participants with the lowest degree of handgrip strength at baseline were significantly more likely to experience cognitive decline in the follow-up period than those with the highest grip strength, who maintained a higher level of cognitive function. Similarly, low handgrip strength was shown to predict the onset of cognitive impairment in a 5-year prospective study of 555 people aged 85 years and over (Taekema et al., 2010).

Unexplained weight loss is a characteristic of both frailty and AD (see Chapter 5, Weight loss and nutritional disorders). Burns and colleagues (2010) examined body composition in a cross-sectional study of 70 older people with early AD compared with 70 matched controls without dementia. After adjusting for possible confounders, they determined that lean body mass was reduced in people with early AD compared with those without dementia, and they suggest that weight loss in early AD may be related to a loss of lean body mass (sarcopenia), as there was no difference in total body fat or percentage of fat values between the groups. In a very large cross-sectional study of body composition in 7105 women aged over 75 years, low muscle mass was associated with cognitive impairment (Nourhashemi et al., 2002). Looking later in the disease process, Buchman and colleagues (2006) showed in a clinical-pathological study of 298 older people that a low body mass index (BMI) before death was associated with a higher level of AD pathology in the brain at autopsy, even in patients without clinical dementia.

## Etiology of frailty in dementia

There appear to be a number of different pathways involved in the development of frailty, and these include the effects of chronic disease, alterations in inflammatory processes, and neuroendocrine and metabolic system changes (Kanapuru and Ershler, 2009). Similar pathways have been implicated in the development of dementia, and AD in particular, with several shared mechanisms of etiology being postulated. Watson and colleagues (2010) suggest there is a shared cerebrovascular pathology underlying motor and cognitive decline, and Raji and colleagues (2010) suggest that raised levels of proinflammatory cytokines such as interleukin-1 and interleukin-6, C-reactive protein, and tumor necrosis factor-alpha (TNF-α), seen in both AD and frailty (Puts et al., 2005), and indicating a state of low-grade chronic inflammation (Zuliani et al., 2007), may be implicated. Chronic inflammation is considered to play a significant role in the pathogenesis of frailty, and high levels of inflammatory markers are associated with the risk of cognitive impairment and dementia, leading to a plausible link between the two states (Avila-Funes et al., 2009). Other possible common underlying mechanisms include decreased energy production at the cellular level, metabolic changes, and oxidative stress (Nourhashemi et al., 2002).

Song and colleagues (2011) have shown that components of a frailty index (Rockwood et al., 2005) that are not known to predict dementia but that do indicate a decline in general health status are able to predict the occurrence of AD and dementia over a ten-year period. They not only hypothesize that the presence of frailty is a risk for developing AD, but also that accumulating any health deficit, including issues not thought to be directly related to dementia risk (such as incontinence, skin problems, deafness, arthritis, or respiratory issues) leads to an increased risk of developing dementia.

The presence of AD pathology (evidenced by amyloid plaques and neurofibrillary tangles) in the brain has been suggested as a possible contributor to the development of frailty. Buchman and colleagues (2008) found a strong association between the presence of frailty before death and the level of AD pathology at autopsy in a study of 165 older people. They felt that frailty may be a noncognitive manifestation of AD, and may be evident before the cognitive symptoms of AD appear. This may be due to the accumulation of the plaques and tangles in neural systems involved with motor function, including the substantia nigra, primary and supplementary motor cortices, and striatum (Buchman et al., 2007).

## Management of frailty in dementia

There is some randomized controlled trial evidence for treatment of frailty using exercise (Binder et al., 2002), but little for the treatment of frailty in dementia. However, it has been suggested that the association between pre-frailty status and cognitive impairment presents an opportunity for preventative interventions with the combined aim of preventing the onset of frailty and slowing cognitive decline (Mhaolain et al., 2011). There is evidence that aerobic exercise may have a disease-modifying effect on AD, by slowing the neurodegenerative processes and promoting neuroprotective neurotrophic factors; thus its use should be considered in all people with dementia (Ahlskog et al., 2011).

Black and Rush (2002) suggest that intervening in functional physical decline may decrease the incidence of cognitive decline, and Rolland and colleagues (2007) have shown that a simple exercise program delivered twice weekly for 1 year to older people with AD residing in a nursing home can reduce the rate of functional decline. Evidence also shows that exercise can improve cognitive function in both cognitively intact (Erickson and Kramer, 2009) and cognitively impaired older people. Exercising aerobically for three 50-minute sessions each week for 6 months delivered a modest improvement in cognition in older people with MCI (Lautenschlager et al., 2008), and Baker and colleagues (2010) have also shown some improved cognitive function in older adults with MCI following a 6-month program of aerobic exercise. In a small study of people with more severe cognitive impairment, Venturelli and colleagues (2011) have shown that regular walking in a group of people with moderately severe dementia can improve walking speed and function in activities of daily living, as well as stabilizing cognitive performance in this group, compared with controls.

It is not clear what type of exercise program should be provided to people with both dementia and frailty. Rockwood and colleagues (2004) noted that resistance exercise decreases serum levels of TNF-α, which is associated with muscle wasting and also with AD. Littbrand and colleagues (2006) have shown that a high-intensity physical-exercise program is feasible in nursing-home residents who are dependent in activities of daily living, irrespective of their cognitive status. In a review of the literature on exercise in dementia, Yu and colleagues (2011) found that aerobic exercise was more acceptable to people with dementia than resistance and balance training exercises, and they suggest that aerobic exercise such as walking should be a core component of any exercise program. Adherence to the program may be a barrier, with poor adherence recognized in some studies (Rolland et al., 2007), thus keeping the program simple is likely to be important.

If frailty can be seen as a vulnerable health state consisting of accumulated deficits (Rockwood et al., 2005), then ameliorating these deficits should also be considered in the management of frailty in dementia. Improving an individual's general health by optimally managing chronic diseases such as diabetes, cardiac failure, or chronic airflow limitation, as well as the detection and management of depressive symptoms, is likely to improve an individual's general health status. If concomitant weight loss has occurred, dietary modification or nutritional supplementation should be considered (Milne et al., 2006) (see Chapter 5).

## Recommendations

1. Consider regular exercise that includes both aerobic exercise such as walking, some resistance/strength training, and balance.
2. Ensure that comorbid medical conditions are recognized and managed optimally.
3. If weight loss and poor appetite are factors in the development of frailty, then the nutritional requirements of the person with dementia should be addressed. Nutritional supplementation may be appropriate.

---

### Case studies

Mrs. U is a 68-year-old woman with mild AD. She lives with her husband, who had become quite concerned about her slow walking and reduced ability to be involved in activities such as gardening, because she had trouble using a spade or lifting small pots. He commented that she had been becoming gradually slower over the previous 5 years, but they had put it down to getting older. Mrs. U said that she felt frustrated that she could not do a lot of the physical things that she wanted to do, and she had trouble getting out of a chair. She was assessed by a physiotherapist, who noted markedly reduced quadriceps strength bilaterally, and reduced upper limb strength. An exercise program was prescribed, which included resistance exercises for both upper and lower limbs, and daily walking. Mr. U was shown how to supervise his wife's exercise program, and she was followed-up by the physiotherapist on several occasions. On review at 3 months Mrs. U was able to stand from a chair without using her arms, and was able to lift her small garden pots. She has continued with her supervised exercise program at least 3 days per week.

Mr. H is an 83-year-old man with moderate dementia living in dementia-specific residential care. He had been gradually losing weight, had become increasingly immobile over the previous 12 months, and had fallen several times when trying to get out of a chair in the dining room. He was assessed by a physiotherapist and found to have generalized lower limb weakness. He was able to cooperate with simple exercises such as chair stands, marching on the spot, and stepping up onto a low block. His family visited regularly and provided some supervision and encouragement to do these exercises. He was also given nutritional supplements twice a day. His weight stabilized over 2 months and he was able to become more active and independent around his room and in the facility. He still required supervision with mobility owing to his impulsiveness, but was now able to go out with his family.

## Key points

- There is evidence that weight loss, decreased muscle strength, and slow walking speed (all features of frailty) antedate the onset of cognitive changes in Alzheimer's disease by many years.
- In large cohort studies with many years of follow-up, more cases of Alzheimer's disease occur in frail older people than in non-frail older people.
- Frailty and dementia may share common underlying mechanisms, including raised levels of proinflammatory cytokines indicating low-grade chronic inflammation, mitochondrial malfunction, and oxidative stress.

## References

Aggarwal, N., Wilson, R., Beck, T., et al. (2006). Motor dysfunction in mild cognitive impairment and the risk of incident Alzheimer disease. *Archives of Neurology*, 63, 1763–1769.

Ahlskog, J., Geda, Y., Graff-Radford, N., et al. (2011). Physical exercise as a preventive or disease-modifying treatment of dementia and brain aging. *Mayo Clinic Proceedings*, 86, 876–884.

Alfaro-Acha, A., Snih, S., Raji, M., et al. (2006). Handgrip strength and cognitive decline in older Mexican Americans. *Journal of Gerontology: Medical Sciences*, 61A, 859–865.

Atkinson, H., Cesari, M., Kritchevsky, S., et al. (2005) Predictors of combined cognitive and physical decline. *Journal of the American Geriatrics Society*, 53, 1197–1202.

Atkinson, H., Rapp, S., Williamson, J., et al. (2010). The relationship between cognitive function and physical performance in older women: results from the Women's Health Initiative Memory Study. *Journal of Gerontology: Medical Sciences*, 65A, 300–306.

Avila-Funes, J., Amieva, H., Barberger-Gateau, P., et al. (2009). Cognitive impairment improves the validity of the phenotype of frailty for adverse health outcomes: the Three-City Study. *Journal of the American Geriatrics Society*, 57, 453–461.

Baker, L., Frank, L., Foster-Schubert, K., et al. (2010) Effects of aerobic exercise on mild cognitive impairment. *Archives of Neurology*, 67, 71–79.

Binder, E., Schechtman, K., Ehsani, A., et al. (2002). Effects of exercise training on frailty in community-dwelling older adults: results of a randomised, controlled trial. *Journal of the American Geriatrics Society*, 50, 1921–1928.

Black, S. and Rush, R. (2002). Cognitive and functional decline in adults aged 75 and older. *Journal of the American Geriatrics Society*, 50, 1978–1986.

Boyle, P., Buchman, A., Wilson, R., et al. (2009). Association of muscle strength with the risk of Alzheimer disease and the rate of cognitive decline in community-dwelling older persons. *Archives of Neurology*, 66, 1339–1344.

Boyle, P., Buchman, A., Wilson, R., et al. (2010) Physical frailty is associated with incident mild cognitive impairment in community-based older persons. *Journal of the American Geriatrics Society*, 58, 248–255.

Buchman, A., Boyle, P., Wilson, R., et al. (2007). Frailty is associated with incident Alzheimer's disease and cognitive decline in the elderly. *Psychosomatic Medicine*, 69, 483–489.

Buchman, A., Schneider, J., Leurgans, S., et al. (2008). Physical frailty in older persons is associated with Alzheimer disease pathology. *Neurology*, 71, 499–504.

Buchman, A., Schneider, J., Wilson, R., et al. (2006) Body mass index in older persons is associated with Alzheimer pathology. *Neurology*, 67, 1949–1954.

Burns, J., Johnson, D., Watts, A., et al. (2010) Reduced lean mass in early Alzheimer disease and its association with brain atrophy. *Archives of Neurology*, 67, 428–433.

Erickson, K. and Kramer, A. (2009). Aerobic exercise effects on cognitive and neural plasticity in older adults. *British Journal of Sports Medicine*, 43, 22–24.

Fried, L., Tangen, C., Walston, J., et al. for the Cardiovascular Health Study Collaborative Research Group (2001). Frailty in older adults: evidence for a phenotype. *Journal of Gerontology: Medical Sciences*, 56A, 146–156.

Inzitari, M., Baldereschi, M., Di Carlo, A., et al. (2007). Impaired attention predicts motor performance decline in older community dwellers with normal baseline mobility: results from the Italian Longitudinal Study on Aging (ILSA). *Journal of Gerontology: Medical Sciences*, 62A, 837–843.

Kanapura, B. and Ershler, W. (2009). Inflammation, coagulation, and the pathway to frailty. *American Journal of Medicine*, 122, 605–613.

Lautenschlager, N., Cox, K., Flicker, L., et al. (2008). Effect of physical activity on cognitive function in older adults at risk for Alzheimer disease: A randomised trial. *Journal of the American Medical Association*, 300, 1027–1037.

Littbrand, H., Rosendahl, E., Lindelof, N., et al. (2006) A high-intensity functional weight-bearing exercise program for older people dependent in activities of daily living and living in residential care facilities: evaluation of the applicability with focus on cognitive function. *Physical Therapy*, 86, 489–498.

Mhaolain, A., Gallagher, D., Crosby, L., et al. (2011). Correlates of frailty in Alzheimer's disease and mild cognitive impairment. *Age & Ageing*, 40, 630–633.

Milne, A., Avenell, A., Potter, J. (2006). Meta-analysis: Protein and energy supplementation in older people. *Archives of Internal Medicine*, 144, 37–48.

Nourhashemi, R., Andrieu, S., Gillette-Guyonnet, S., et al. (2002). Is there a relationship between fat-free soft tissue mass and low cognitive function? Results from a study of 7105 women. *Journal of the American Geriatrics Society*, 50, 1796–1801.

Puts, M., Visser, M., Twisk, J., et al. (2005). Endocrine and inflammatory markers as predictors of frailty. *Clinical Endocrinology*, 63, 403–411.

Raji, M., Al Snih, S., Ostir, G., et al. (2010). Cognitive status and future risk of frailty in older Mexican Americans. *Journal of Gerontology: Medical Sciences*, 65A, 1228–1234.

Rockwood, K., Hogan, D., MacKnight, C. (2000). Conceptualisation and measurement of frailty in elderly people. *Drugs & Aging*, 17, 295–302.

Rockwood, K., Howlett, S., MacKnight, C., et al. (2004). Prevalence, attributes, and outcomes of fitness and frailty in community-dwelling older adults: Report from the Canadian Study of Health and Aging. *Journal of Gerontology: Medical Sciences*, 59A, 1310–1317.

Rockwood, K., Song, X., MacKnight, C., et al. (2005). A global clinical measure of fitness and frailty in elderly people. *Canadian Medical Association Journal*, 173, 489–495.

Rolland, Y., Pillard, F., Klapouszcak, A., et al. (2007). Exercise program for nursing home residents with Alzheimer's disease: a 1-year randomised, controlled trial. *Journal of the American Geriatrics Society*, 55, 158–165.

Samper-Ternent, R., Al Snih, S., Raji, M., et al. (2008). Relationship between frailty and cognitive decline in older Mexican Americans. *Journal of the American Geriatrics Society*, 56, 1845–1852.

Song, X., Mitniski, A., Rockwood, K. (2011). Nontraditional risk factors combine to predict Alzheimer disease and dementia. *Neurology*, 77, 227–234.

Taekema, D., Gusselkloo, J., Maier, A., et al. (2010). Handgrip strength as a predictor of functional, psychological and social health. A prospective population-based study among the oldest old. *Age & Ageing*, 39, 331–337.

Venturelli, M., Scarsini, R., Schena, F. (2011). Six-month walking program changes cognitive and ADL performance in patients with Alzheimer. *American Journal of Alzheimer's Disease and Other Dementias*, 26, 381–388.

Waite, L., Grayson, D., Piguet, O., et al. (2005). Gait slowing as a predictor of incident dementia: 6-year longitudinal data from the Sydney Older Persons Study. *Journal of the Neurological Sciences*, 229–230, 89–93.

Wang, L., Larson, E., Bowen, J., et al. (2006). Performance-based physical function and future dementia in older people. *Archives of Internal Medicine*, 166, 1115–1120.

Watson, H., Rosano, C., Boudreau, R., et al. for the Health ABC Study. (2010). Executive function, memory and gait speed decline in well-functioning older adults. *Journal of Gerontology: Medical Sciences*, 65A, 1093–1100.

Yu, F. (2011). Guiding research and practice: a conceptual model for aerobic exercise training in Alzheimer's disease. *American Journal of Alzheimer's Disease and Other Dementias*, 26, 184–194.

Zuliani, G., Ranzini, M., Guerra, G., et al. (2007). Plasma cytokines profile in older subjects with late onset Alzheimer's disease or vascular dementia. *Journal of Psychiatric Research*, 41, 686–693.

# Index

acetylcholine, age-related decrease, 67
activities of daily living (ADL), 86, 89, 90
aerobic exercise, 114–115
age-related macular degeneration (AMD), 87
age-related sleep patterns, 74
Alzheimer's disease (AD)
    aerobic exercise benefits, 114–115
    dental caries, 100
    dysphagia, 46
    energy requirement increase, 45
    epilepsy as risk factor, 32
    falls association, 5, 7
    frailty, 112, 113, 114
    gait impairment, 5
    inflammation role in development, 101, 113–114
    late-onset, delirium in, 16
    prediction, from frailty index, 114
    seizures, 30–31, 32, 34
        pathogenesis, 33
    sleep disturbances, 74, 75, 76
    urinary incontinence, 62, 63
    visual dysfunction, 86
        pathophysiology, 86, 87–88
        symptoms/types, 90, 91
    visual hallucinations, 91
    visual variant (VVAD), 88
    visuospatial dysfunction, 90
    weight loss and malnutrition, 40, 42
        causes, 43–45
        nutritional supplementation, 47–48
amyloid plaques, in retina, 88
amyloid precursor protein, 33
anterior cingulate cortex (ACC), 45
anti-epileptic therapy, 34–35, 102
antimuscarinic drugs, 66–67

antipsychotics, 22, 33, 102
apathy, 43, 44, 101
ApoE4 allele, 43, 76
arthritis, 47
attentional skills, delirium management, 22
axonal sprouting, 33

behavioural disturbances
    in delirium, 19
    falls associated, 7
    impact on oral health, 101
    weight loss and malnutrition, 44–45
benzodiazepines, 6, 22
bladder
    normal control/physiology, 61–62
    overactive, 61, 66–67
body mass index (BMI), 47, 113
brain structural changes, weight loss
        and, 43, 45

CADASIL, 88
carer stress/mental health problems, 80
carers, burden of
    oral health problems, 101
    sleep disturbances, 80
    urinary incontinence, 67–68
    weight loss, 43
case studies
    delirium, 23
    epileptic seizures, 35–36
    fecal incontinence, 70
    falls, 10–11
    frailty, 115–116
    oral disease, 106–107
    sleep disturbances, 81–82
    urinary incontinence, 69–70

visual dysfunction, 93–94
  weight loss and malnutrition, 52
cholinergic deficiency, 17
cholinesterase inhibitors, 33
  falls associated, 7
  sleep disturbances and, 76
  urinary incontinence and, 66
  weight loss and malnutrition, 46
circadian rhythm changes, 74, 76, 77
cognitive impairment
  exercise program benefits, 114–115
  falls associated, 3, 4
  frailty association, 111, 112
  mild *see* mild cognitive impairment
  visual acuity problems, 89
colour vision impairment, 91
community
  activity programs, 79
  fall reduction/prevention, 9
  prompted voiding program, 66
comorbidity, 1
  in dementia, literature search, 1–2
Confusion Assessment Method (CAM), 20, 22
constipation, 61, 68
continence, 60–61, 63–64
  *see also* urinary incontinence (UI)
continence aids, 67
contrast sensitivity, 88–89
Creutzfeldt–Jakob disease (CJD), 32, 88, 90

dawn dusk simulation (DDS) light
    therapy, 77
daytime sleepiness, 75–76
delirium, in dementia, 15–24
  assessment, 20–21
  case studies, 23
  clinical features, 15, 18, 19–20
  definition, 15
  dementia cause/effect relationship, 16–17
  diagnostic difficulties, 18, 20
  epidemiology, 15–16
  etiology, 16–17
  impact on dementia, 15, 18–19
  management, 21–22
  mortality, 18
  pathogenesis, 17
  persistent, 15, 18, 20
  prevention, in hospital, 21
  recommendations, 22–23
  risk and risk factors, 15, 17–18, 19
Delirium Room, 21
dental caries, 99, 102
  epidemiology, 100, 101
  medications impact on, 102

dental hygiene/care *see* oral health;
    oral hygiene
dental plaque, 99
dentistry, 105
  minimal intervention, 105
dentures, 99, 100, 106
detrusor hyperactivity, 61, 66–67
diarrhea, 61
dietary intake, alterations, 43–44
  *see also* malnutrition
diffuse Lewy body disease (DLBD)
  delirium *vs* dementia, 19
  gait impairment and falls, 5, 7
  neurovascular instability, 6
  seizures, 31–32
  urinary incontinence, 63
donepezil, 66
Down syndrome, seizures, 32
drugs *see* medications
dual-tasking, 6
dysphagia (swallowing difficulties), 43, 46
  management/interventions, 50

Eating Behaviour Scale, 47
eating environment, 48–49
eating patterns, disordered, 43–44, 45
education of staff, 48
  delirium management, 22
  dental hygiene, 105
  falls prevention, 8–9
  nutritional supplementation, 47, 48
energy
  increased requirements, 45
  intake, timing, 49
enteral feeding, 50–51
  hand feeding *vs*, 51
environmental factors, nutritional intake
    improvement, 48–49
epileptic seizures (and epilepsy), 30–36
  in AD *see* Alzheimer's disease
  case studies, 35–36
  definition, 30
  diagnosis, 34
  epidemiology and prevalence, 30–32
  etiology, 33
  falls associated, 35
  features, 34
  management, 34–35
  recommendations, 35
  risk and risk factors, 31, 34
  as risk factor for dementia, 32–33
  seizure types, 31, 34
  in specific dementias/conditions, 31–32
  treatment (drugs), 34–35

exercise programs
  delirium incidence reduction, 21
  fall prevention, 9
  frailty and cognitive decline reduction, 114–115
  prompted voiding program with, 65–66

falls, in dementia, 3–11
  assessment, 8
  behavioural disturbances, 7
  case studies, 10–11
  definition, 3
  dementia pathology and, 5, 6
  epidemiology, 3–4
  etiology, 4–5
  gait impairment, 5
  management, 8–9
  medication effects, 6–7, 9
  preventative interventions, 8–9, 10
  recommendations, 10
  risk and risk factors, 3, 7, 8
  seizures associated, 35
  sequelae/effects, 3, 4
fecal impaction with overflow, 61, 68
fecal incontinence, 61, 68
  case study, 70
  epidemiology, 62
  management, 68
  prevalence, and risk factors, 68
feeding, enteral see enteral feeding
feeding behaviour changes, 44
fibre (dietary), intake, 68
finger foods, 49
food(s)
  familiar, and familiar environment
      for, 48–49
  finger, 49
  refusal, 44
  types, to improve eating/nutrition, 49
frailty, 111–116
  case studies, 115–116
  causes, 111
  definition/criteria, 111, 112
  epidemiology, 111–113
  etiology, 113–114
  management, 114–115
  as noncognitive feature of AD, 114
  recommendations, 115
frontotemporal dementia (FTD)
  dysphagia, 46
  eating pattern changes, 43–44
  urinary incontinence, 63–64
  weight loss and malnutrition, 40
functional incontinence, 61

gait
  impairment, 5
  normal, 5
  see also walking
gingival hyperplasia, 102
glucose metabolism, 45

haloperidol, 21, 22
handgrip strength, decreased, 113
hemispatial neglect, 91
hip fractures, 4, 19, 21
hippocampal lesions, falls and, 5
hospitalization
  after falls, 4
  delirium precipitation, 16–17, 18
  delirium prevention, 21
  protein/energy intake reduced,
      interventions, 50
Huntington's disease, seizures, 32
hyberbolic state, 45
hypotension, orthostatic (postural), 6

incontinence, 60–70
  see also fecal incontinence; urinary
      incontinence (UI)
incontinence pads/aids, 67
individualized social activity interventions
      (ISAI), 79
indwelling catheter (IDC), 67
inflammation, 101, 113–114

lean body mass, reduced, 113
levetiracetam, 35
light therapy, 77
  melatonin with, 78

macular retinal nerve fibre layer, 87
macular volume, reduction, 87
malnutrition, 40
  assessment, 47, 51
  behavioral symptoms
      associated, 44–45
  case studies, 52
  causes/pathogenesis, 41, 42–46
  dementia impact, 40–42
  disordered eating patterns, 43–44
  dysphagia, 46
  intervention and management, 46, 47–51
  in nursing home residents, 41
  recommendations for management, 51–52
  see also weight loss
meals, 49–50
medial temporal lobe, abnormalities, 45

medications
    falls associated, 6–7, 9
    impact on oral health, 102–103
    seizure threshold reduced, 33
    for sleep disturbances, 77–78
    for urinary incontinence, 66–67
    weight loss/malnutrition association, 46
melatonin
    delirium management, 22
    sleep disturbance intervention, 78
mild cognitive impairment (MCI)
    frailty and reduced motor function,
        112
    retinal nerve fibre layer, 87
    sleep pattern changes, 75, 81–82
Mini Nutritional Assessment (MNA), 47
mouthwash, 104
multitasking (dual-tasking), 6
muscle strength decrease, 111, 113

nasogastric tubes, 50
National Institute of Clinical Excellence,
        delirium diagnosis, 20
neurofibrillary tangles, 75
neuroleptics, falls associated, 6
neurovascular instability, 6
night monitoring system (NMS), 80
nursing homes and residential care
    malnutrition in, 41
    oral hygiene and dental care, 105
    urinary incontinence prevalence, 62
    visual impairment, 92
nutritional disorders see malnutrition; weight
        loss
nutritional state, dementia impact, 40–42
nutritional supplementation, 47–48, 50

optic flow, impairment, 91
optic nerve, changes, 87
oral disease, 99–107
    assessment, 104, 105
    case studies, 106–107
    epidemiology, 100
    management, 103
    symptoms and signs, 103
    treatment, 104–105
oral health
    behavioural changes impact, 101
    benefits, 99
    goals, 103–104
    impact of dementia on, 100–102
    medication impact on, 102–103
    recommendations, 106

oral hygiene
    daily care recommendations, 104, 106
    poor state, 99, 100
    staff education on, 105
oral ulceration, 102
orthostatic hypotension, 6
oxybutynin, 66–67

Parkinson's disease
    dysphagia, 46
    gait impairment and falls, 5, 7
    neurovascular instability, 6
    urinary incontinence, 63
pelvic floor exercises, 66
perceptual disturbances, 19
percutaneous endoscopic gastrostomy (PEG)
        tubes, 50–51
periodontal disease, 102
physical activity
    increased nutritional intake, 50
    sleep disturbance management, 79
    see also exercise programs
physical restraints, fall prevention, 9
polysomnography, 76
postural hypotension, 6
prompted voiding (PV) programs, 65–66
    design and goals, 65
    outcome and resource requirements,
        65–66, 68

REM sleep, decrease, 75, 76
residential care see nursing homes and
        residential care
respite care, 80
restlessness, night time, walking impact, 79
retinal nerve fibre layer (RNFL), thickness, 87
risperidone, 78

saliva, reduced, 102
saliva stimulators, 106
sedation, in dentistry, 105
sedatives, 77
seizures see epileptic seizures (and epilepsy)
sialorrhea, 102
sleep
    age-related changes, 74
    deprivation in carers, 80
sleep disturbances in dementia, 74–82
    carer burden, 80
    case studies, 81–82
    epidemiology, 75–77
    intervention and treatment, 77–79
    pathology, 74–75

sleep disturbances in dementia (*cont.*)
  recommendations, 81
  types, 76
stress incontinence, 61
sucking reflexes, 102
sundowning, management, 22
swallowing problems *see* dysphagia
synaptic hyperactivity, 33

'talking while walking' test, 6
teeth
  low number, dementia association, 101
  preservation, benefits, 105

urge incontinence, 61
urinary incontinence (UI), 8, 60–70
  assessment, 64
  caregiver burden, 67–68
  case studies, 69–70
  causes, 60, 63, 64, 66
  definition, 60
  dementia types and, 62, 63–64
  epidemiology, 62
  impact of dementia on, 63–64
  intervention and management, 64–68
    continence aids, 67
    medications, 66–67
    PV program *see* prompted voiding (PV)
      programs
  prevalence and increase in, 60, 62
  recommendations, 69
  stress incontinence, 61
  types, 61
urinary obstruction with overflow, 61

vascular dementia
  delirium in, 16
  gait impairment and falls, 5
  urinary incontinence, 62
  weight loss and malnutrition, 40
visual acuity impairment, 89, 91
  recommendations, 92
visual dysfunction, 86–94
  assessment, 87, 92
  case studies, 93–94

definition, 86
features/types, 88–91
impact in dementia, 88
interventions, 93
pathology, 86–88
recommendations, 92, 93
in residential care, 92
types of visual problem, 86, 88
visual field defects, 86, 89–90
visual hallucinations, 88, 91–92
visual motion, optic flow impairment and, 91
visuospatial dysfunction, 90

walking
  impact on nighttime restlessness, 79
  speed decrease, frailty, 111, 112
  *see also* gait
wandering, falls and, 7
weight
  dementia impact on, 40–42
  gain, 42, 46
weight loss, 40–53
  assessment, 47, 51
  behavioural symptoms and, 44–45
  case studies, 52
  causes/pathogenesis, 41, 42–46
    cholinesterase inhibitors, 46
  dietary intake alterations, 43–44
  disordered eating patterns, 43–44
  epidemiology and prevalence, 42
  frailty and, 113
  increased energy needs, 45
  intervention and management, 46,
    47–51
      education of staff, 48
      enteral feeding, 50–51
      environmental factors, 48–49
      multifactorial strategy, 49–50
      nutritional supplementation, 47–48
      targeted approaches, 49–50
  preceding dementia, 41–42
  recommendations for management, 51–52

xerostomia (dry mouth), 99, 100, 101
  drugs causing, 102

Printed in the United States
By Bookmasters